W9-BZE-182

INTUITIVE

REIKI

For Our Times

INTUITIVE
REIKI

For Our Times

ESSENTIAL TECHNIQUES
FOR ENHANCING
YOUR PRACTICE

AMY Z. ROWLAND

Healing Arts Press
Rochester, Vermont

Healing Arts Press
One Park Street
Rochester, Vermont 05767
www.HealingArtsPress.com

Healing Arts Press is a division of Inner Traditions International

Copyright © 2006 by Amy Zaffarano Rowland

All rights reserved. No part of this book may be reproduced or utilized in any form or by any means, electronic or mechanical, including photocopying, recording, or by any information storage and retrieval system, without permission in writing from the publisher.

Note to the reader: This book is intended as an informational guide. The remedies, approaches, and techniques described herein are meant to supplement, and not to be a substitute for, professional medical care or treatment. They should not be used to treat a serious ailment without prior consultation with a qualified health care professional.

LIBRARY OF CONGRESS CATALOGING-IN-PUBLICATION DATA

Rowland, Amy Zaffarano.
  Intuitive reiki for our times : essential techniques for enhancing your practice / Amy Z. Rowland.
     p. cm.
  ISBN-10: 1-59477-099-9
  ISBN-13: 978-1-59477-099-9
  1. Reiki (Healing system)   I. Title.
  RZ403.R45R66 2006
  615.8'51—dc22

                                                    2006008703

Printed and bound in the United States

10   9   8   7   6

Photographs of Albert Seaman and Iryna Zhyrenko by Connie Bell-Dixon.
Photographs of Reiki Masters Laurelle Shanti Gaia by D.; William Lee Rand by Michael Schoepholtz; Mari Hall by Sonja Whitfield; and Linda Schiller-Hanna by Kim McBryde.

Text design by Peri Champine
Text layout by Virginia Scott Bowman
This book was typeset in Berkeley Oldstyle with Amadeus, Calligraphic, Bulmer, and Benji Modern as the display typefaces

To send correspondence to the author of this book, mail a first-class letter to the author c/o Inner Traditions • Bear & Company, One Park Street, Rochester, VT 05767, and we will forward the communication.

This book is dedicated, with love and gratitude, to my teacher, Reiki Master Beth Gray, and to my mother, Rita Maria Zaffarano . . .

CONTENTS

ACKNOWLEDGMENTS

Reiki continues to be the greatest blessing of my life. As a soul, I am grateful now and always to all those who have taught me Reiki and who continue to teach me Reiki, to the loving community of Reiki practitioners and teachers that spans the globe and, again and again, touches my heart, and to the energy itself, which has brought so much healing to those I love and to me. I am thankful for a deeper knowledge and love of Spirit, for a greater appreciation of my innate healing ability and my intuition, enhanced by Reiki, and for all my life experiences with Reiki.

No words can describe the value that I place on the guidance given to me by my Reiki "ancestors," Mikao Usui, Chujiro Hayashi, and Hawayo Takata, as I do Reiki. I bow to my teachers of traditional Usui Reiki, Beth Gray and Frank DuGan, and to my teachers of Usui Reiki Ryoho and Gendai Reiki, Tom Rigler and Hiroshi Doi. The kindness and wisdom of Hyakuten Inamoto and Dave King have profoundly affected me, and the dedication, hard work, and generosity of spirit of Tom Rigler, Rick Rivard, and Andrew Bowling, who sponsored Hiroshi Doi's first visit to the West, will always inspire me. I honor those within the Usui Reiki Ryoho Gakkai who have allowed information about Reiki's history and techniques, as they have been taught in Japan, to be shared with Reiki practitioners around the world.

Reiki itself teaches us all, and as we share the stories of our experiences with Reiki, we learn from one another. This book, which contains so many stories, has offered me the opportunity to learn from my fellow Reiki Masters and practitioners. In particular, I would like to thank Yvonne deVastey, Robert Fueston, Laurelle Shanti Gaia, Mari Hall, Linda Schiller Hanna, janeAnne Narrin, Frank Arjava Petter,

William Rand, and Linda Urie for their willingness to be interviewed about Reiki and intuition. Lauren Bissett, Peter Conver, Lynn Deemer, Mani Evanko, Candace Ferrandino, Michael Fischer, Terry and John Graybill, Natalie James, Glenda Johnson, Carole Koch, Colleen Lavdar, Leslie Levy, Dana Limpert, Robin McAteer, Daniel O'Hara, Ann Pedersen, Noreen Ryen, Barbara Sautter, Doris Scherer, Connie Seneko, Kay Sivel, Lynn Thiel, and Rose Troilo allowed me to describe their experiences in classes, in client sessions, at Reikishares, and facing the crises of daily life. To all of you—and to all of those whose names are not revealed but whose shared experiences enriched this book—my heartfelt thanks.

Albert Seaman and Iryna Zhyrenko, dear Reiki Master friends and the models for the photos in the book, thank you for being willing to give of your time and your energy to help to make the practical techniques described in the text clear and helpful. Connie Bell-Dixon, I appreciate the crisp, clear photographs you've taken, the years of comforting friendship you've given, and the invite to a dazzling island vacation to help me relax and get my second wind. Paula Heller, your willingness to transcribe an interview, and Terry Graybill, your help with labeling the photos and tagging the manuscript proved essential to completing the book. I am grateful to you all.

It is unlikely this book would ever have been written without a few special Reiki friends playing angels and creating opportunities for me to come together with others of like mind and interest. Jeanne White, thank you for introducing me to the local chapter of AHNA. Gail Buletza, thank you for inviting me to be your guest at the A.R.E. conference on Intuition Development, where I first heard Linda Schiller Hanna and Mary Roach speak. Sandra Franklin, thank you for inviting me to do a book signing at Celestine, where I connected with so many wonderful people who have become students, friends, and colleagues. You made sure that I met William Rand, whose interest in an article for *Reiki News Magazine* on the intuitive Reiki techniques I had learned from Beth Gray prompted me to write a tribute to her and the article that inspired this book.

Those Reiki practitioners and teachers who receive my e-mailed requests for distant healing, sent on behalf of so many in need, thank you for the healing you sent my way to help me bring this book to its conclusion—and thank you for all you do, day after day, to bring Reiki healing into this world: Dave Bause, Karen

Biehl, Sajeda Bhallo, Shirley Brack, Barbara Brand, Phyllis Butler, Jim and Linda Chokas, Nadine Chudoba, Sheila Corrao, Joann and John Davis, Patricia Duffy, Leslie Ellis, Martin Evans, John Hako, Barbara Friling, Vincent Green, Tina Marie Houseweart, Judy Jurgaitis, Deborah Keough, Linda Killian, John King, Carol Klekotka, Cheryl Beth Kuchler, Janet Kuchler, Denys Lapping, Nancy Leaming, Amy Levin, Marianne Liberto, Mary Anne Macko, Eileen Morgan, Norman and Dolores Merrell, Catherine McGinley, Colleen Nicholas, Becky Pierotti, Laura Porter, Sharon Riegner, Wendy Robb, Claudia Rydel, Lauren Sage, Betty Sheridan, Karen Thompson, John Van Trieste, Frank Vicente, Ann Woolsey, Anastasia Wilson, Diane Zielinski. My thanks also to all of my Reiki students, especially those who have attended a Reiki and Intuition Workshop and helped me to focus and refine some of the material for this book. Although you think of me as a teacher, I always learn so much from you.

Donna Davidson and Scott Pruyn of the Dreamcatcher in Skippack; Denys Lapping of Earth Angel in East Greenville; and all of those who have hosted Reiki classes I have taught and Reikishares I have coordinated, I appreciate your willingness to make space available for spiritual pathwork of all kinds.

Fred Even, Donna Fasano, Ellen Philips, Ann Reid, thanks for encouraging me as a writer. Your insights and advice have been invaluable, your kind words just what I needed to keep me going page after page, chapter after chapter.

Susan Davidson, my editor at Healing Arts Press, thank you for your sharp eye and your wise perspective. Your helpful suggestions, gently offered, have made *Intuitive Reiki for Our Times* a better book. Thank you for your patience, your integrity, and dedication—and your kindness. I feel grateful to the publisher and to everyone on the editorial staff at Healing Arts Press for sharing a commitment to excellence that is expressed not only in the quality of the books you publish, but also in your support of your authors. I am so glad to be one of them!

Finally, thank you who are reading this now for being willing to *listen* not only to the Reiki energy in your hands, but to your own inner wisdom, which has guided you to pick up this book and browse through its pages or buy it and bring it home to your own bookshelf. May you find within these pages much that brings you healing and instruction, and much that enlightens and entertains. May you discover here the story of your own soul and its voice, *listen* to it, and hear it resonate as true.

INTRODUCTION: BRIDGE OF LIGHT

Reiki is holistic, healing the whole person. Yet few people ever ask themselves what it would be like to feel truly whole, truly well. Most of us are too focused on seeking symptomatic relief from tension headaches or aching backs or sore feet to allow ourselves to imagine what it would be like to experience radiant physical health, mental clarity, emotional happiness, and spiritual well-being. When we do imagine, it is the sense of spiritual well-being that seems most elusive.

As children, most of us enjoy a natural sense of being protected, comforted, loved, guided, and connected to all of life. Yet by the time we are adults many of us have forgotten that state of grace through the numbing effect of repeated blows: an unexpected death of a close friend or family member, the loss of a job, the heartache of rejected love, the disappointment of not being chosen, acknowledged, valued. Our self-esteem suffers, and we feel battered and dull, insecure, anxious, isolated, confused. Yet we think we are no better off, nor any worse off, than our friends and family and colleagues. "Life is hard," we read, on the bumper sticker of the van stuck in traffic in front of us, "and then you die."

Then we learn Reiki. We begin to heal from old injuries. We start to feel relief from chronic symptoms that have plagued us for years. We start to recognize that we are not responding to stress with the same sense of helplessness. We are becoming resilient. We are beginning to lighten up, finding joy and accepting the possibility that there might be more to life than we thought not so long ago.

We take pleasure, too, in offering to do Reiki for others. We are so glad to be able to help, to soothe, to comfort. We become grateful. We become, more and more often, kind.

And one day, as we sit in meditation or in the meditation-like altered state of doing Reiki, listening to the energy flowing through our hands, something flashes into our awareness with such intensity that we see it behind our closed eyes: an explosion of light; a gentle swirl of color; a crystal clear image of a mother's face, full of tender love, as she reaches for her child. Or we recognize the scent of the sea, though we are several hundred miles inland, in a room with closed windows. Or we hear a refrain from a song, though we are doing Reiki without background music playing. Or we hear a voice, as Hawayo Takata did, with our inner ears. Somehow, we know something new, something more, something of value, without knowing how we know.

This moment in time can mark the beginning of a greater sense of spiritual well-being, if we are able to recognize it for what it is: a fleeting perception of oneness with the source of universal life-force energy. Some might call this source God or Spirit or Divine Mind, described across religions as all-present, all-powerful, all-knowing. Others may prefer to call this source universal consciousness or, simply, a higher power. By whatever name we call this source, when we are immersed in the flow of universal life-force energy we can perceive across apparent physical boundaries that we normally take for granted as solid and "real," and we can glimpse events beyond the conceptual barriers we habitually observe between past, present, and future.

It is during just such moments that Spirit "drops in" and leaves us a calling card. Imagine this invitation hand-lettered in gold on the finest parchment paper: "You are invited to a celebration of the union of your individual soul with the divine, to take place on this very day, and again and again and again, from this day forward. The honor of your conscious presence is requested. Please R.S.V.P."

If we accept the invitation, we are on our way to being restored not only to physical, mental, and emotional health and happiness, but to spiritual well-being: to a childlike sense of grace, of being divinely protected, guided, comforted, and loved. And if we refuse? No matter. In time another such invitation will be issued. Spirit can wait. Spirit has all eternity.

Fortunately, committed Reiki practice makes it quite likely that another invitation to acknowledge this conscious connection to the divine will come soon. Those who learn and practice Reiki often find themselves witnessing physical healing in their clients that is far beyond their intellectual understanding and their clients' physicians' best hopes. This is one way Reiki invites us to acknowledge this source. Another occurs when a Reiki practitioner receives intuitive impressions during a treatment. Practitioner and client both may find themselves afterward reflecting on how such a connection is possible. Is there some truth in the message of the sages that "we are one"?

But intuitive guidance may also come to Reiki practitioners at other times, away from the Reiki table. Such guidance might comes in dreams, in a daydream, in meditation, in a sudden moment of insight—and sometimes for no apparent reason at all.

REIKI GUIDANCE IN A DREAM

"Yes, I understand Reiki works, but *how* does it work?"

In 1994, shortly after I began teaching Reiki and hearing that question from beginning Reiki students again and again in more or less the same words, I had a dream that offered me an answer.

In the dream, I was in a video store at a local shopping mall browsing through the boxes of movies available for sale. Behind me and all around me, I could hear the owner and the other customers in conversation about their work. As I strolled nearer to the checkout, the owner asked me, "And what do you do?"

I had been thinking about how I would answer if I were asked this question, and I responded with the answer I had rehearsed in my mind: "I teach and practice Reiki, a holistic healing method and a form of bodywork and energy medicine."

"Reiki?" The owner grunted. "Well, I've never heard of it. You say that it is a holistic healing method? There are a lot of those now. How is it different from all the rest?"

"Well," I said, hesitating, as I searched for words. "Other holistic healing

3

methods teach the mind. The practitioner must learn to focus and concentrate the mind to form an intention so that the healing energy will be transferred to the client. The practitioner might use visualization or recite an affirmation or say a prayer to focus this intention to bring healing. Reiki doesn't require that kind of mental discipline. Reiki doesn't teach the mind."

I continued, now with confidence. "Reiki teaches the soul, and the soul instantly recognizes its nature and its source—and rejoices. The soul is infused into the physical body, so the body accepts Reiki. The mind, on the other hand, thinks and analyzes and attempts to make logical order of this experience. So the mind may struggle for weeks or months or years with questions about Reiki: What is it? How does it work? Why does it work? This thinking and analyzing can go on long after the practitioner has learned Reiki and used it many times with good results. Eventually these questions become like background noise, and the practitioner lets them go or gives up asking them, because the answers no longer seem important."

I woke up, stunned by the wisdom of my dream self. "Reiki doesn't teach the mind. Reiki teaches the soul." As I sat up in bed and rubbed sleep from my eyes, I could feel my understanding shifting, become clearer and more comfortable. Of course, Reiki teaches the soul. Now I had an answer for those students who came to class wanting to satisfy their intellectual curiosity, wanting to problem solve the mystery of Reiki.

In the many Reiki classes that I have taught since that morning, whenever I have felt that it would be appropriate and helpful to do so I have shared the story and the message of this dream, to allow others the benefit of its guidance.

INTUITION: VOICE OF THE SOUL

Dreams, meditations, and intuition often do provide answers to questions, solutions to problems, direction in periods of uncertainty. This was the case for Hawayo Takata, the first Western Reiki Master, whose ability and willingness to recognize and honor the voice of the soul guided her to complete recovery of her health and fulfillment in her life's work as a healer and spiritual teacher.

Some Reiki practitioners, like Takata, come to Reiki by making a choice to listen to their inner guidance; many more think their decision to learn Reiki is logical and practical, and that intuition plays no part in their decision. Yet most Reiki practitioners soon realize that intuition has an important role to play in client treatments and self-treatments, offering guidance and direction and supporting deeper, more complete healing.

Because accidents, injuries, and illness that affect the physical body are often occasioned by stress or trauma or occur as an accompaniment to depression, understanding the mental, emotional, and spiritual causes for these conditions is usually necessary for complete healing. This understanding can be obtained in many ways. Some people find the inner strength to face the past and forgive those who caused them pain by creating artwork, writing in a journal, doing dreamwork, going for counseling, speaking out in support groups, or undergoing hypnotherapy or psychoanalysis. Reiki-trained health care and service providers frequently recommend these methods to their patients and clients to support emotional and mental healing. Often, however, even such conscientious efforts are not enough to bring complete release. Something more is needed: an intuitive impression that comes into a Reiki practitioner's mind during a treatment, promptly offered to the client to interpret and understand, can be the tool that unlocks the door to the hidden causes of physical discomfort and makes possible complete healing.

Consider the many Reiki practitioners in many occupations who would like to be more intuitive in order to better help their clients: a health care worker daydreams about developing the skills of a medical intuitive; a veterinarian's assistant admires television's "pet psychic" and wishes to become a proficient animal communicator; a beautician yearns to know exactly the right words to comfort one of her regulars who is going through a difficult time; a pastoral counselor desires a more spiritually guided connection to his clients; a geriatric nurse hopes to get an inner prompting that will enable her to be at the bedside of a dying patient too weak to press the "call" button, to comfort him as he passes on; a wildlife rehabilitator wants to understand how best to support the recovery of an injured bird of prey; a psychotherapist seeks insight into a traumatized client's past in order to create an effective guided visualization for her emotional healing. On some level all these practitioners are aware that a strong intuitive connection to their clients will support deeper and more lasting healing.

INTUITION IN REIKI HEALING

Reiki, in bringing healing on all levels of being, beckons its practitioners gently, gradually forward on the path toward spiritual enlightenment. Just as we are naturally healing, so we are naturally intuitive—born with a direct connection to Spirit and some level of awareness of our inner guidance. When we learn Reiki, that connection to Spirit becomes clearer, steadier, stronger, and our awareness of that connection becomes ever more conscious. We sense it in the flow of healing energy in our hands and in the surprising insights that come to mind, more and more often, for our Reiki clients and for ourselves.

Sadly, most Reiki practitioners are not taught to expect to receive such insights as they do Reiki, nor are they taught how to recognize, value, and communicate these insights. Learning more about intuition and how and why intuitive impressions arise as we do Reiki can help a practitioner become a more effective channel for healing. This can bring the practitioner a sense of joy and being in harmony with the soul's purpose that is beyond the satisfaction of service or the peace of meditation.

The history of Reiki provides strong evidence of the value of intuition. While most Reiki practitioners are not taught to use intuitively guided techniques as they do Reiki hands-on or distant healing, there are a few traditional lineages in the West that do encourage receptivity to intuition.

In Japan, within the Usui Reiki Ryoho Gakkai, the organization that offers instruction in the Reiki method, a practitioner must master a technique called Reiji-ho, "allowing Reiki to guide you to a healing place," in order to progress from beginning to more advanced levels. This technique (presented in detail later in this book) is a form of advanced scanning in which the practitioner asks to connect to the Reiki energy and to be shown intuitively which areas of the body need healing; the practitioner follows this guidance, again and again, until the treatment is complete. Mastery of this technique, which often takes several years, also requires the practitioner to arrive at an accurate diagnosis of the client's condition and to predict how many Reiki treatments will be needed to bring about a cure. While such a requirement would be discouraged in the West (because it is illegal for anyone without a medical license to diagnose or prescribe), the fact of its existence is more evidence of the strong foundation that Reiki provides for developing intuition.

Another demonstration that Reiki supports intuitive development (for practitioners in all lineages) is to be found at Reikishares, or healing circles. Anyone observing practitioners from both traditional and nontraditional lineages at the bodywork tables will see some of them quite naturally and comfortably, and others more hesitantly, sharing the intuitive impressions they have received with those they are treating.

In the Reiki classes I teach, I have welcomed practitioners trained in other lineages; they have been able to learn to receive intuitive impressions as they do Reiki, even though this is not the way they were originally taught. At the Reiki and Intuition workshops that I have taught in the last few years, the same holds true: when practitioners make an effort to open up to the possibility of receiving intuitive impressions in support of healing, they can learn to recognize and understand this guidance without discarding it because of self-doubt or distorting it because of fears or desires; and they can learn to relay guidance received for a client with gentleness and humility, in harmony with Spirit, without attachment to results.

How is it that such practitioners are able to become more receptive to intuition and more skilled in sharing the impressions they receive? A commitment to Reiki practice is a commitment to self-healing and to bringing healing to others. This is pathwork that Spirit honors and rewards. That flash of intuitive insight is a blessing: it enlightens and empowers the practitioner and client both, in keeping with the nature of Reiki itself. For Reiki practitioners, intuitive development occurs naturally as we heal and grow spiritually through our practice; indeed, becoming intuitive may even be integral to our further spiritual development. To listen to our intuition is to listen to our inner teacher, to our inner wisdom, to the voice of the soul. To listen to our intuition is to accept Spirit's invitation to recognize and accept, again and again, that we are loved, protected, and guided by the divine.

1

INTUITION IN REIKI HISTORY

The story of Mikao Usui's pilgrimage to the top of Mt. Kurama outside Kyoto, Japan, and his twenty-one day fast, meditation, and prayer vigil prior to receiving the great light and healing energy of Reiki, is taught to students of Reiki worldwide. Perhaps this is so that this gentle, spiritual man will never be forgotten, and perhaps this is so that we will appreciate how quickly and easily we are able to receive Reiki, even though Mikao Usui dedicated years of his life to his spiritual quest before enlightenment. Or we may retell his story so often because it is a good story that speaks to us on many levels and resonates as truth.

The history of Reiki begins with Mikao Usui and his search for greater wisdom, but it does not end with him: it quickly becomes the history of many dedicated teachers and students, many committed practitioners, many healing hands. Today, Reiki is practiced by millions of people around the planet, with more learning and receiving Reiki healing every day.

While many of the details of Mikao Usui's life are still unknown, we now have a clearer understanding of Reiki's beginnings, thanks to the efforts of several contemporary Reiki Masters. German Reiki Master and author Frank Arjava

Petter's work has included on-site research in Japan, translating the text of Mikao Usui's memorial stone at Sahoji Temple and, more recently, the manual Usui gave to his new students. American Reiki Master William Rand has visited Japan, corroborated Petter's research, and publicized accounts of his travels. Reiki Masters Rick Rivard of Canada, Tom Rigler of the United States, and Andrew Bowling of the United Kingdom sponsored the first visit of a Japanese Reiki Master, Hiroshi Doi, to the West in 1998. The cultural exchange that began then has continued and expanded, with other Japanese Reiki Masters joining Doi-Sensai to present workshops at Usui Reiki Ryoho International conferences, attended by Reiki Masters from all around the world.

All of these individuals must be acknowledged for their courage and generosity of spirit. Through their willingness to share their knowledge and experiences of Reiki across lineages and national borders, they have brought much-needed healing to a world that still suffers from the spiritual wounds of religious, racial, social, economic, and class discrimination and intolerance.

The impact of this healing is uplifting to individual and global consciousness: in acknowledging that the essence of Reiki transcends its many variations, those who practice and teach are empowered to reach out to one another in friendship and in shared service. We take a step closer to world peace.

This is a truth that Hawayo Takata, who learned Reiki in the 1930s, when the world was on the brink of World War II, must have understood, for when she taught Reiki to her own students she taught many different techniques. While she has been criticized for this pedagogical method, it is possible to consider her actions in another light: perhaps Takata was guided by an inner wisdom to teach the techniques that would be most appropriate and helpful to her students in each class.

In fact, Takata's ability to listen to her inner guidance and act upon it allowed her to play a key role in the history of Reiki, bringing it from Japan to the island of Hawaii, from where it spread throughout the world. The story is familiar to many Reiki practitioners. When Takata was in her early thirties, newly widowed and faced with the responsibility of raising her young children alone, she became so ill that she was advised to have surgery. As she lay on the operating table, resting with her eyes closed and waiting for the procedure to begin, she heard someone say, quite distinctly, "No, there is another way."* She opened her eyes and looked around the room, but there was no one in it but herself. She decided she must have imagined the voice. She rested her head back down on the table and, once more, closed her eyes. The voice spoke again: "No, there is another way." This time when she opened her eyes and looked around, she saw nurses bustling about, making preparations for her surgery. None of them were even looking in her direction. Again, she lay down and closed her eyes. Once more she heard the voice giving her the same message. Once more she raised herself up to survey the room.

By now the surgeons were busy scrubbing up and donning surgical gowns and gloves. She asked if any of them had spoken to her. None of them had. Then she asked if any of them knew of an alternative method of treating her condition that might allow her to avoid the surgery. The chief surgeon told her then that he had heard of a clinic in Tokyo run by a Japanese physician named Chujiro Hayashi; the clinic was becoming well known for the remarkable recoveries of its patients.

When Hawayo Takata heard this news she decided to listen to the advice of the mysterious voice that only she had heard: she refused the surgery, left the hospital, and made arrangements to go to Japan and receive treatments at Hayashi's clinic. Under Hayashi's care she was completely cured, and under Hayashi's instruction she learned Reiki and eventually became the first Western Reiki Master.

Yet consider the self-doubt that Takata must have suffered as she lay on that operating table, hearing a voice with no apparent source. At first she dismissed it as her imagination. Because she heard it yet again—and then again—she finally determined that she would listen and act upon it: she gathered her courage to challenge the surgeons and nurses preparing to operate upon her: could there be any other way for her to recover her health? When the chief surgeon men-

---

*I write this story about Takata as I recall Reiki Master Reverend Beth Gray telling it to my class in March 1987 and to later classes at which I assisted between 1987 and Beth Gray's retirement from teaching Reiki in 1992. Reiki Master Helen Haberly, another student of Takata's, reports the same story in a slightly different version in her book, *Reiki: Hawayo Takata's Story*. She quotes the voice Takata heard as saying, "The operation is not necessary."

tioned the only other option that came into his mind, Takata trusted that this was the way she must explore. How difficult it must have been for her to refuse the operation, to discharge herself from the hospital, and to pack her bag for a journey to an unknown clinic in Japan in hope of a cure, simply because she had heard an inner voice.

Takata's willingness to be guided by her intuition led her to her teacher, Chujiro Hayashi, a physician, retired naval officer, and Reiki Master trained by Mikao Usui himself and asked by Usui to establish a Reiki clinic in Tokyo. At Hayashi's clinic, Takata was treated with Reiki again and again until all her physical ills were completely cured. Pleased with her experience of Reiki and with the outcome of all the treatments she received, Takata decided she wanted to learn Reiki and to bring this healing method back with her to the island of Hawaii, where she would establish a center where more people could come to receive Reiki healing. She made several trips to Japan over the course of the next few years, sometimes staying for extended periods of time, so that Hayashi could teach her Reiki. Eventually Takata asked Hayashi to teach her to the Master level, so that she could teach those who came to her center who wanted to learn Reiki themselves.

In her diary, in an entry dated May 1936, she wrote:

> What was more than pleasing was that Mr. Hayashi has granted to bestow upon me the secret of Shinpiden—Kokiyu-Ho and the Leiji-Ho—the utmost secret in the Energy Science . . . imagine my happiness to think that I have the honor and respect to be trusted with this gift—a gift of a life time. I promised within me to do my utmost in regard to this beautiful and wonderful teaching that I just received . . . to do what is right thru sincereness [sic] and kindness . . . and shall regard and respect the Teaching and its Teacher with utmost reverence.*

---

*Although I originally accessed this diary entry in summer 2005 on the web at reikihistory. topcities.com/Takata.html, this website is no longer posted; an alternate website that posts this and other entries from Takata's diary is James Deacon's www.geocities.com/fascin8or/reiki_takata_ diary.htm. In addition, physical copies of selected pages from Takata's diary, including this one, continue to be passed down by some Usui Reiki Masters trained in the Western tradition.

Thanks to the on-site research and international cultural exchange regarding Reiki history and practices in recent years, we now know that Shinpiden is the name used to describe the master level of training. The first of the two techniques Takata mentions in her diary entry is most probably Koki-ho, offering Reiki healing through the breath; this technique is not associated with any particular level of Reiki training. The second, which she writes as "Leiji-Ho," is Reiji-ho, connecting to the Reiki energy intuitively to receive inner guidance regarding the course of treatment. This guidance may describe the sequence of hand positions to be used during an individual session, and it may also suggest diagnosis and recommend the number of Reiki sessions necessary for the client to be cured.

This information comes to us courtesy of Japanese Reiki Master Hiroshi Doi, who has visited the West several times to share information about the Japanese tradition of Reiki. According to Doi-Sensai, both the Koki-ho and Reiji-ho techniques have been taught and practiced in Japan since the time of Mikao Usui through the Usui Reiki Ryoho Gakkai, the learning society established by Usui's students around the time of his death in 1926 to continue the teaching of Reiki. Mastery of the Reiji-ho technique is required of Reiki practitioners before they are permitted to progress from Shoden (entry) to Okuden (deep mystery) teachings.

Yet Takata regarded learning these two techniques as "the secret of Shinpiden . . . a gift of a life-time." Could it be that Hayashi taught Takata Reiki techniques in a different sequence than the sequence used by the Gakkai? This is certainly possible, since Hayashi himself had separated from the organization and taught independently. It is likely that he mentored Takata in a gentle, supportive way, as the Gakkai does with all who learn Reiki. If so, he would often have watched her at the treatment table and noticed her perception of the Reiki energy in her hands becoming more subtle as she continued to practice. The ability to feel *hibiki*, energy resonance or vibrations in the hands, is one of the prerequisites for learning Reiji-ho; the other is learning to scan the body with the hands. When the practitioner develops proficiency in sensing energy in the hands and scanning the body, then the master may teach Reiji-ho. It is very likely that this is how Hayashi taught this technique to Takata.

Why did Takata regard these two techniques in particular as so precious? Perhaps Reiji-ho was rarely taught to her fellow students at Hayashi's clinic, and she was aware of this. Even today, within the Usui Reiki Ryoho Gakkai, it is considered a difficult technique, often taking many years to master. (The criteria applied are quite stringent: the practitioner must demonstrate the ability to be guided intuitively by the Reiki energy to perform client treatment, to accurately diagnose the client's condition, and to predict the number of Reiki sessions needed for the client to be cured.) As a result, many students stay at Shoden (entry) level of Reiki for a long time before progressing to Okuden (deep mystery) level. In May 1936, Takata was certainly Okuden level; perhaps, since she mentions Shinpiden, Hayashi was beginning to prepare her to teach. Chujiro Hayashi signed a statement certifying Takata to teach on February 21, 1938; this statement was filed in the city and county of Honolulu, Hawaii on the same date.

Takata's path to Reiki required that she overcome her self-doubt and listen to an inner voice. A few years later, when she was completely healthy and committed to Reiki practice and teaching, Hayashi taught her a Reiki technique that required her to allow the Reiki energy to guide her intuitively. Perhaps, with the passage of time and the hindsight that her intuition had once guided her rightly, this was an easy technique for her to learn. As far as I know, it is not a technique that she passed along to most of her Reiki students—even her Reiki Master students—as it has traditionally been taught in the Usui Reiki Ryoho Gakkai. Instead, Takata taught intuitive Reiki techniques to only a handful of her Reiki Master students.

Nor did she teach them all in the same way. My teacher for Reiki I and II, Usui Reiki Master Reverend Beth Gray, worked as a professional clairvoyant prior to learning Reiki. I believe that Hawayo Takata tailored the attunements and instruction she gave to Beth, at all levels, to accommodate her psychic gifts; perhaps Takata foresaw that those students who would be drawn to Reiki Master Beth Gray would themselves be interested in developing their intuition and using it in Reiki healing.

REIKI ENHANCES INTUITION

During 1987, I took both Reiki I and II classes with Reverend Beth Gray. For someone whose intuitive guidance seemed on-again, off-again, it was good news to hear that the repeated Reiki attunements received in the Reiki I class would enhance intuition. We could begin to expect to receive intuitive impressions as we worked hands-on—perhaps not often at first, but more often as we continued to practice Reiki. This ability, we were told, would become even more pronounced with the additional attunements we would receive in Reiki II class.

During Reiki II, much of our training focused on working with intuition. Beth explained that we have an internal set of senses that corresponds to our external senses. We can receive an impression in the form of sight, sound, smell, taste, or touch; an impression can come as a wash of feeling; or we can simply "know" without knowing how we know. The second symbol, which most practitioners call the mental-emotional healing symbol, Beth also called the talking symbol. By using this symbol we could "talk" to our clients through the Reiki connection. Beth encouraged us to be polite, to introduce ourselves by name, to ask our clients, "How are you?" and "Are there any areas in particular you would like treated with Reiki today?"

What might follow these simple questions, asked in the silence of the practitioner's mind, could be slowly forming, simple impressions; sudden flashes; a two-way dialogue; or a one-sided monologue, in which the client floods the practitioner with words, images, or other kinds of impressions. Or silence might follow the asking of these questions. The practitioner offers Reiki healing, but the client always has free will to accept or reject it, on whatever level it is offered: physical, mental, emotional, spiritual. We would have distant-healing clients who were communicative and clients who wanted only to rest, relax, and absorb the Reiki energy. Whatever the client's choice, we were to offer Reiki without judgment and with unconditional love.

There would also be clients whose communication to us was unclear and confusing. Should that occur, we might ask for clarification. Whatever impressions we did receive we were to present to the client, if appropriate, without attempting to interpret them. Receiving intuitive impressions as we did Reiki, we would learn, was like dreaming someone else's dream. As with all dreams, the original dreamer is the one most likely to understand the meaning.

This particular intuitive Reiki technique was dreamlike in another way: just

14

as in dreams, the subconscious mind will only reveal to consciousness what is ready to be processed—or, in this case, healed—in some way. Practitioners who were concerned that this technique might be an invasion of the client's privacy found this clarification reassuring and felt even more compelled to present impressions they received, with compassion.

She also reminded us that past, present, and future are all one to Spirit, and therefore, to the Reiki energy. Impressions could come from any of these points in what we think of as chronological or linear time. If we were unsure whether the impression we were receiving presented a past event, a present concern, or a future possibility, we were to ask for additional guidance.

In the months and years that followed my Reiki classes with Beth Gray, I was schooled by the energy itself in the validity of these points. Although I usually closed my eyes as I did hands-on and distant healing, I often saw both fragmentary and coherent images with my third eye.* As I did Reiki I also saw words on this mental screen, and I read and understood their meaning. I heard voices and music with my inner ear. I smelled fragrant summer flowers in the middle of winter and dirty diapers in a house without babies. I learned to sense the feelings of my client without being overwhelmed by them. And many times, though I was open to receiving impressions as I did Reiki, I saw only a luminous darkness and felt content to watch the energy of Reiki as light, at peace.

NIAGARA FALLS, UNITED STATES—CANADIAN BORDER, SEPTEMBER 2002

Despite the fact that my mother was seriously ill, I knew that I must make the trip to Toronto in late September 2002, to attend the Fifth Usui Reiki Ryoho

---

*Located just above the center point between the eyebrows, this is the same area of the brain where we visualize a scene unfolding as we read a book or tell a story, listen to a sports game on the radio, or daydream. With our eyes closed and our attention focused, this area becomes a softly lit theater where our mind can show us "movies" of our own or Spirit's choosing.

International Conference. I also knew that it was important that I take advantage of the conference presenters' invitation to arrive a day early and spend time touring with Japanese Reiki Masters Hiroshi Doi and Hyakuten Inamoto, their translators, and other early bird conference guests. Tom Rigler, who had taught me the Usui Reiki Ryoho techniques to the Shinpiden level in classes in Pennsylvania and Maryland, would be there; and I wanted to meet Rick Rivard, with whom I had corresponded by e-mail for years.

The highlight of the preconference day was a visit to Niagara Falls, which included a ride on a tour boat called *The Maid of the Mist*, which chugs slowly around in the churning waters at the base of the falls. On board, donned in oversized transparent raincoats, Reiki Masters from Japan, Canada, and the United States stood together talking about Reiki even as they smiled up at the falls in wonder. Despite the differences in cultural backgrounds and personal philosophies, despite the differences in teaching methods, we had come together in friendship. The next day we would attend the Usui Reiki Ryoho International conference, some of us as presenters, some of us as very willing students, eager to learn more of Reiki's history and traditional and modern Japanese Reiki techniques.

Standing shoulder to shoulder with another Reiki Master, wondering aloud about Mikao Usui's life, I was struck by the beauty of the clouded sky above the falls, almost golden-white with the light of the hidden sun. I felt a tremendous happiness. The sense of harmony, of rightness, in being on board *The Maid of the Mist* with so many new Reiki friends from around the world was profound, and also strangely familiar.

Over the next few hours, as we continued playing tourists, I struggled to make sense of my feeling of *deja vu*. Then I recalled a dream I had recorded on waking a few years earlier: my parents, older relatives, and friends of the family were gathered in the boarding area of an airport, chattering with excitement about the trip they were about to take. Could I go along? I wanted to know. Wherever they were going, I was sure, was a wonderful place.

They began to board. I moved to the end of the boarding line. My Aunt Francis, looking pretty and prepared in her traveling clothes, offered me a consoling smile. "You can't come on this trip, dear," she said. "It's not your time."

Dismayed, I watched her turn away and disappear through the door into the plane's skyway. Then, in the nonlinear way of dreams, I was granted a glimpse of the plane's destination. As if I was inside the airplane's cockpit looking out through the wide span of its window, I saw a beautiful white cloud, mottled with golden light; it felt vast, deep, forever.

Then I awoke. *Heaven*, I thought, as I reflected on the dream that morning over my coffee. I felt sad. I knew I would be missing many loved ones soon. I also felt comforted. They were all going into that amazing light.

On *The Maid of the Mist*, with other Reiki Masters from around the world who had set aside their differences to share their knowledge freely out of their love for Reiki, I had seen the same sky. Hours later my mind fit the puzzle pieces together of experience and dream: *heaven on earth*. For me, in that moment, alive with an awareness of the unity I felt with my Reiki companions, this was one of the potentials of Reiki realized: peace, harmony, healing energy flowing all around, heaven on earth.*

Reiki's potential for world healing is acknowledged—indeed, it is forecast—within the long inscription on Mikao Usui's memorial stone at Sahoji Temple, translated by Frank Arjava Petter and Chetna M. Kobayashi in *Reiki Fire*. It says: "If Reiki can be spread throughout the world it will touch the human heart and the morals of society. It will be helpful for many people, and will not only heal disease, but the Earth as a whole."

Reiki now unifies many people around the world in healing practice, service, and spiritual pathwork. Intuition's role in Reiki history, its importance to Takata's healing and spiritual journey, its use in some traditionally taught Reiki techniques in the West and in Japan, is an invitation to all Reiki practitioners and teachers to reflect on its value in their own lives and to commit to learning how to work with intuition in Reiki practice. Perhaps it will not only help us and those we love and care for to heal more completely and permanently. Perhaps

---

*Reiki historians will be aware that the 2002 Usui Reiki Ryoho International Conference ended with some behind-the-scenes dissension. After five years of sponsoring this event at locations around the world, Rick Rivard and Tom Rigler retired as conference organizers and hosts; the 2003 Usui Reiki Ryoho International Conference, hosted by Reiki Masters in Silkeborg, Denmark, was the last of its kind. Since then, however, both Hiroshi Doi and Hyakuten Inamoto have made several trips to the West to teach master classes and to continue the cultural exchange.

Reiki will help us to heal the deeper wounds of the world and come together in greater harmony and hope.

SUGGESTIONS FOR PRACTITIONERS

Consider the possibility that Hawayo Takata, who was willing to honor her inner guidance by traveling from Hawaii to Japan in pursuit of complete healing and who treasured her teacher's instruction in the technique of Reiji-ho, the intuitive placement of hands, was guided throughout her Reiki practice and teaching career. Does this make it any easier to understand her teaching methods? Takata, who taught variations in techniques, in symbols, and in attunements to her students and to the Reiki Masters she initiated, has been widely criticized. Could it be that Takata was listening to an inner guidance that helped her to envision a world that would need to be reminded that it is not the form, but the essence, of Reiki that brings healing, enlightenment, and empowerment?

NOW YOU

If you know a practitioner whose training is different from your own, consider talking to her about what brought her to Reiki. See if her path parallels or overlaps your own. Ask her about how she views her Reiki practice. Is her understanding radically different from your own, or do you have common ground? Ask her about some of her experiences with Reiki. Share some of your experiences. Rather than standing apart, guarding your differences, can you build a bridge of Reiki light between you that will allow you to connect in friendship and love?

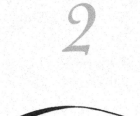

INTUITION AT
A REIKI CLASS

Our culture acknowledges the importance of touch for healthy development and for healing, so some fortunate students come to their first Reiki class already confident of the innately healing abilities of their hands. Learning Reiki feels familiar and comfortable to them, a welcome expansion of a skill they are glad to possess. Many other students who come to class lacking this confidence soon learn that healing through touch is easy to do when clearly discernable sensations of healing energy—the result of the Reiki attunements—flow through their hands to guide them. Generally, by the end of the class session all of the students are quite capable of distinguishing subtle changes in Reiki's healing energy through their hands; they are also excited at the prospect of being able to offer effective healing to others and to themselves.

In contrast, our culture has a history of doubting the value of intuition, psychic powers, and extrasensory perception—and in some eras has ridiculed or condemned outright those who claimed such abilities. During the last decade, the public has shown much more interest in intuitive development (as evidenced by the popularity of TV shows such as John Edward's *Crossing Over* and books by Sylvia Browne, Laura Day, Mona Lisa Schulz, and others). However, there are still few people who feel confident of their intuitive abilities as they sit in their first Reiki class.

Reiki enhances this natural ability—a prospect that does not appeal to every student, as the story that follows illustrates.

BEGINNINGS

One beautiful Saturday morning in July, at the start of a Reiki I class, I invited my two students to tell me about themselves and how they came to Reiki.

Doris, a tall, young woman in her mid-twenties with blue eyes, a shoulder length fall of brown hair, and a bright smile warming her face, told us that during the last year she had experienced some serious health problems for the first time in her life. She had sought out Reiki practitioners, somehow knowing that their hands would bring her healing and relief. Now she wanted to learn Reiki herself, so that she could offer it to friends and family.

"What about giving yourself some Reiki each day?" I asked. "Wouldn't you like to be able to do that?"

She looked at me in astonishment. "Will I really be able to do that? You mean I can give Reiki to myself?"

I nodded.

Her smile widened into a grin. "Cool!" she said, with happy enthusiasm.

I turned to my other student, a middle-aged woman named Rose, whose blue eyes and fair hair reminded me of her sister Robin, whom I had come to know well in the last year as she worked to complete her Reiki Master training. Rose's face, like Robin's, hints at her Irish-American ancestry. Both, as it turns out, are what the Irish call "a wee bit fey"—intuitive—each in their own way.

"What about you, Rose? Have you experienced Reiki?" I asked.

She nodded. "Robin has worked on me several times, and she has sent me distant healing, too, when I needed it." Rose became reflective for a moment, then added, almost shyly, "I've been practicing Native American healing. I find it really interesting." She paused, then added, "I've been doing meditation every day."

20

"Good for you!" I said. "I'm glad that you've been exploring and that you are meditating. That's a discipline, a real commitment to your own spiritual path."

I looked from Rose to Doris. "Do either of you have any questions you would like answered right away?"

Doris looked serious. "I do. I have some questions. I would like to make sure that I understand correctly how Reiki works. I've asked a couple of the practitioners who worked on me about it, and they said that doing Reiki won't drain me or make me feel physically tired. Is that true?"

"Yes, that's true," I said. "When you do Reiki, you channel or serve as a conduit for universal life-force energy. As you practice Reiki more and more, you become increasingly sensitive to the energy that comes into you and flows through you. Sometimes you can actually feel Reiki energy coming into you from above—through your head and upper body—and then out from your heart, through your shoulders, down your arms, and through your hands into your client. And sometimes," I said, smiling, "you will feel that path of energy flow even when you are the client, and you are treating yourself."

"Really?" she asked, her eyes wide.

"Yes," I said. "I want you to understand, though, that once in while, as you do a Reiki treatment, you may also feel energy coming up through the soles of your feet, or from above and below, or from all around you. It is 'universal life-force energy'—it comes from the universe through you in whatever way will best serve the client's needs. So, to answer your question, when you do Reiki you won't feel tired or drained after a treatment, because you are tapping universal life-force energy, rather than your own physical energy."

Doris settled back in her chair, beginning to look reassured.

"In fact, whenever you do a Reiki treatment, you receive some healing, too," I added.

"The practitioners who worked on me mentioned something about that."

"Let me give you an analogy. Doing a Reiki treatment on a client is a lot like watering a garden with a garden hose. In the hands of a good gardener, the plants and the ground in which they are planted get a thorough soaking every time the gardener waters the garden, and the inside of the garden hose gets wet too. Because of the water that flows through it, the hose stays flexible, and that helps to make the garden hose last. So when we work on a client, the client receives *most* of the healing energy, but because the energy streams through us on its way to the client, we receive some healing benefits too: we become calmer, more relaxed, and feel a greater sense of well-being."

Doris looked pleased. "That sounds good to me!"

Rose nodded. "That's what Robin told me. That's one of the reasons I want to learn Reiki."

"I have another question," Doris said, looking almost embarrassed.

"That's okay! Please ask away."

"I've already tried to use my hands to do Reiki. My grandmother has been so ill, and I really wanted to help her. I asked another Reiki practitioner to work on her, and my grandmother relaxed and went to sleep. After that I placed my hands on my grandmother in the same way as the practitoner—and my hands got hot! Was that okay?"

I laughed. "Of course. I think you were inspired!"

She looked at me quizzically.

Rose spoke up suddenly. "I tried to do Reiki, too. I put my hands on my abdomen in the same positions Robin used to see what it would feel like. I think my hands felt a little bit warmer."

"Well, there is certainly nothing wrong with trying out the hand positions," I said, to reassure them both. "Consciously or not, you know that touch is healing, and you have given yourselves a chance to learn how you can work with intention to increase that quality of healing."

I glanced from one to the other. "I want to tell you also that sometimes, in the days and weeks before a Reiki class, the energy 'drops in' to say hello. It's not uncommon for new Reiki students to tell me that they have felt sensations of energy in their hands or around the top of their heads."

They shared a look of gleeful surprise. Their expressions reminded me of children at a birthday party who have just learned that there will be not only cake and ice cream and presents, but balloons and party favors, too.

"Reiki is *universal life-force energy,* but that's not the only way the word can be translated from Japanese. Reiki also means 'Spirit' or 'soul-guided energy.' So perhaps," I said, focusing on Rose, "Spirit decided to visit you in advance of the class to prepare you and to give you a sense of what the energy will usually feel like in your hands." I turned to Doris. "And perhaps the Reiki energy came to answer your soul's call to help your grandmother make her transition."

She nodded, and a touch of sadness dimmed the light in her face for a moment, like a thin cloud obscuring the sun.

Doris and Rose are fairly typical of people who decide to learn Reiki. Doris described "somehow knowing" that receiving Reiki treatments would relieve her pain and help her recover from the serious health problems she had been experiencing, yet on the day that she walked into the Reiki class, she was unaware that she would be able to use Reiki on herself. Like many people she had been guided to Reiki, but she didn't really know much about it.

Rose, on the other hand, had been actively exploring her own spirituality. Because of her focus on Native American healing, she had started to train herself to read and reflect on "signs" in nature that other people, less aware, might ignore: sighting a hawk soaring high overhead, a mouse scurrying through her garden, a butterfly fluttering across her path. She also gave careful attention to the imagery of her dreams and to any ideas that came to her during her meditations. She was alert for seeming coincidences that occurred in her daily life and did not dismiss them, but gave them serious consideration. When someone from her immediate family stepped forward to offer her Reiki, she was ready to be open to the experience, accept the healing, and claim Reiki as a spiritual tool by signing up for a class herself.

Both Doris and Rose listened to their inner guidance to help them make the decision to learn Reiki. Doris mentioned "somehow knowing" Reiki would help her feel better, but, as of the start of the class, she hadn't reflected on the reason for this intuitive knowing. Rose was offered Reiki and encouraged to take the class by her older sister, who has often served, over the years, as an external source of guidance and advice. For Rose, who asks for guidance in prayer and meditation each day, saying, "Yes, I want to learn Reiki," was an easy decision.

The Reiki energy "visited" both Doris and Rose in advance of the class. While this certainly doesn't happen to every student, a surprising number report feeling fleeting sensations of energy, usually in their hands, before their first class. For some this serves as a confirmation of guidance already heeded; for others it provides validation that the direction chosen is in accord with the wisdom of the soul. For Doris and Rose, their brief experiences of the energy in their hands before the class provided comfort and healing. This beckoned them forward, like a light up ahead on a dark path, guiding and illuminating the way.

Yet Doris still felt afraid of the shadows, as her next question revealed.

ß

Doris's face brightened again as she smiled. "You said that you don't mind questions. . . ."

"No, not at all. Go ahead," I said, encouraging her to free herself of any remaining concerns.

"Is learning Reiki going to make me able to know what is going to happen in advance—or make me see ghosts or spirits?"

I was taken aback. I took a long, steadying breath and began to think about which question to answer first. Then she gave me a clue.

She shuddered and shook her head forcibly. "I really don't want to see ghosts or spirits."

"No," I said. "You won't see ghosts, if you don't want to see ghosts." I smiled in sympathy. "I'm like you. *I* don't want to see ghosts either, not even in the movies. I sat through *The Sixth Sense* with my eyes closed half the time! Whenever the little boy saw the specter of one of those gory murder victims, I wanted to run out of the theater!" I laughed. "God knows I am a complete coward when it comes to seeing ghosts, so I don't see ghosts—and I never have."

She looked relieved.

"To be honest with you, though, I must tell you that since learning Reiki I have become much more sensitive to energy, so there have been times when I have felt the presence of a ghost or spirit. But it hasn't been a frightening thing. I've been able to pray and send Reiki to help one ghost cross over to the other side and go to the Light; and sometimes I sense my mother around me—she died in 2004—and that's actually a comfort. I think that is a fairly common experience, too, for people to sense the presence around them of a loved one who has passed on." I gave her a reassuring smile. "But God knows I don't want to see ghosts, so I don't see them!"

Doris still looked concerned. "What about knowing something in advance? I had an experience once that really scared me. I was driving my car, cruising along a road, and all of a sudden I just stopped the car. Then another car whizzed across the road in front of me, inches in front of my bumper. I was terrified!"

"Would you have been killed if you had continued driving?"

"Yes," she nodded, looking almost ashamed.

"So listening to that inner guidance to stop the car saved your life?"

"Yes," she said, "but the whole experience scared me. How did I know to *do* that?"

"Do you believe in God?"

"Yes."

"Do you believe that God is all-knowing?"

"I suppose so. . . ."

"Then perhaps God just gave you a heads up—a message—and because you listened, you are alive today."

She nodded thoughtfully.

"Reiki does enhance intuition, just as it enhances the natural ability that we all have to bring healing through touch. Have you ever noticed a pregnant woman standing with her hands nested over her belly, comforting her unborn child? Or have you reached for your knee when you've fallen on it to ease your own pain?"

"Sure," she said. "Everybody does that!"

"It's just natural, isn't it? But what is our nature? People of most religions believe that human nature contains some element, some spark, of the divine. Perhaps the ability to bring healing through touch allows us to feel the source of compassion in ourselves, and perhaps our intuition—our inner knowing— connects us to the source of all knowing, even if only for a moment. Does that make sense?"

Doris nodded.

"Intuition is our very own internal navigation system—it's been called the compass of the soul—and it helps us find our way in life: find our purpose, find our happiness, and find our spiritual path, our way home to God."

Doris's smile warmed her eyes. She gathered her courage and asked another question. "So being intuitive doesn't have to be a scary thing?"

I shook my head. "No, in fact, for many people receiving an intuitive impression is a lot like dreaming. Do you ever remember your dreams?"

"Yes, sometimes."

"Have you ever noticed that the images we see and the sounds we hear in dreams seem to play like a movie on an inner screen right *here*?" I asked, touching the area of my forehead just above and between my eyebrows.

"Sure."

"Yogis call this area the third eye, and they use it as a focal point for meditation. When you or I dream or daydream, we see with this inner eye. When artists imagine paintings or authors imagine scenes for books, they are seeing with this inner eye—even though they may have their external eyes wide open at the same time. It is this inner, spiritual eye that opens and sees when we receive a 'flash' of intuition."

Doris listened intently.

"My Reiki teacher, Reverend Beth Gray, told her students that we all have a set of inner senses that correspond to our external senses of sight, hearing, smell, taste, and touch. We even have special names for some of these inner senses—*clairvoyance* for inner vision, *clairaudience* for inner hearing, and *clairsentience* for inner knowing. I think that's what you experienced when you knew you had to stop your car suddenly without knowing why. Your willingness to pay attention to that inner knowing probably saved your life."

"Will Reiki definitely make me more intuitive?"

"Reiki will open the door to your inner life. It will be up to you to decide when you want to walk through that door."

REIKI PRACTITIONERS GRADUALLY BECOME MORE INTUITIVE

For most practitioners, becoming more intuitive is something that occurs gently and gradually, over time. If they are traditionally taught, they learn to listen to their hands for guidance on how long to stay in each position as they do a treatment. This is a wonderful discipline: besides giving the client a thorough, effective treatment, it teaches the practitioner to focus inner awareness on subtle energy. With continued practice, this awareness becomes more and more refined —and the energy teaches us some fascinating lessons.

For example, a practitioner might know, without knowing how he knows, where the Reiki energy is flowing in his client's body as it flows away from his hands. Or a practitioner may feel as if her hands have disappeared and become pure energy. Or a practitioner might feel as if his hands have merged with the client, because the sense of physical separateness has been suspended; or the client may describe the sensation of feeling the practitioner's hands still in place, flowing with healing energy, even after the practitioner has moved to the opposite end of the table. Such perceptions of the Reiki energy invite the practitioner and the client to realize that we are "One in Spirit"—and in the flow of Reiki. In that unity it becomes possible, even easy, to connect to Spirit to receive intuitive impressions that can be of help to the client. It also becomes easier to receive clear guidance for ourselves.

INTUITION SUPPORTS HEALING
AND SPIRITUAL GROWTH

When I learned Reiki in 1987, and was told by my teacher that it would enhance my intuition, I did not understand what the value of this "enhanced intuition" might be. I thought it could be helpful to have some clue as to the original cause of a client's illness or condition, but I could not guess in what other ways it would be of benefit. Now, after many years of practice, I recognize that intuitive impressions received during a Reiki session provide healing guidance of several different kinds.

Sometimes they do provide insight into the original cause of "issues in the tissues," enabling the client to identify suppressed feelings that may be causing tension or stress or contributing to disease; sometimes they provide a clue to the event or situation that triggered those suppressed emotions, whether it occurred long ago, in the recent past, or is still ongoing. (When this kind of impression comes up, the client may have quite a lot of work to do—remembering, reflecting, releasing—to complete the emotional and mental healing process. Much of this work will necessarily be done outside the Reiki treatment room, after the close of the session. Practitioners may want to suggest journaling or other creative work, or pastoral counseling, psychotherapy, or group therapy to clients who want to actively engage in this process and continue it to completion on their own or with the aid of professional mental health care providers. Such a commitment will make deeper, more lasting healing possible on all levels.)

Intuitive impressions received by a practitioner during a Reiki session and shared with the client can also prompt the client to make a decision about medical treatment or a healthy lifestyle change. Sometimes they encourage the client to communicate with family members, friends, or coworkers, extending healing beyond the setting of the Reiki session into the individual's private or professional sphere. Occasionally these Spirit-guided impressions offer the client comfort, confirmation, and hope for the future.

SUGGESTIONS FOR PRACTITIONERS

Perhaps you learned Reiki last week or last month; perhaps you were certified so long ago that you do not remember the details of what occurred in class. Claim a quiet place and time to think about your path to Reiki—a place that you can revisit often as you read this book.

If you are a regular commuter, you may want to use a relaxed hour or so of your ride time (with radio or CD player and cell phone off) for these reflections. A quiet room in your home where you are able to retreat and close the door to interruptions may also be adequate for this review. Better than ride time or a quiet room is a space dedicated to contemplation or service: a room used for meditation or for Reiki can work well. You may also find sanctuary in a space where you can connect to nature: some people make a habit of visiting a particular bench in a park or a grassy spot beside a stream. There, they sit down and relax and watch—and watching outwardly, also look inward.

Walking along familiar roads, literally retracing the steps of other years, can also bring the past vividly to mind. Those with access to a labyrinth may choose to walk it in a moving meditation, spiraling slowly to the center and back as they contemplate their path to Reiki. Some of you will want to record your discoveries as you retrace your history and claim its hidden gifts. The moving point of a pen is an excellent single-point focus for this journey, for it is an external object that moves across the blank page only when guided by your hand and directed by your mind and heart. Trust it to take you where you need to go to recollect the treasures of the past, even if you are housebound and without any other form of transportation.

NOW YOU

Settled into your safe space? Good. This is only a first foray into memory, so let it be brief—just a quick look back to see what comes to mind easily.

Your first task is this: identify the person, place, or thing (newspaper or magazine article, book, website, business card, brochure, flyer, tee shirt) that first presented the name Reiki to you. If you learned Reiki recently, this task may be easy. If you learned years ago, expect to spend longer remembering (literally "re-membering": recalling an experience to make it part of you and your conscious awareness once again). Of course, if you have become deeply committed to Reiki practice you may have considered this question in the past and your answer—or answers—are ready.

Whether or not you complete this first task with effort or with ease, please take time afterward to practice gratitude. Be thankful for those individuals and circumstances that came together in your life to encourage you to learn Reiki and to enjoy the benefits of healing and spiritual transformation that it brings. By allowing yourself to live the central Reiki principle, "Just for today, be grateful," you deepen your awareness of the energy and open your heart to greater blessings, already on their way.

Your second task is one of self-discovery through reflection. As you explore recent memory, consider how you think about the past. Do you see visual images as you remember? Or is it the voices of people in conversation or the music playing in the background that you recall? Then think further back in time to an early family celebration—a birthday party or a holiday dinner. Can you easily recall the scent of smoke lingering in the air after the birthday candles were blown out, or the aroma of the pumpkin pie that baked in the oven wafting through the house? Check yourself against a more recent memory: popcorn at the movies, a cup of cappuccino at a coffee shop, hot dogs with mustard at a baseball game.

The ability to identify the sense that dominates your memories gives you a strong clue as to how intuition is most likely to work for you. This same inner sense may be the first that you notice as you begin to do intuitive Reiki. Your daydreams and visions of the future are another. When you think about where you want to go next year for vacation, do you picture the place in your mind? Or do you find yourself imagining the sounds or the smells? For example, if you are planning on going to a beach, do you think first about the deep blue of the ocean under a cloudless sky? Or do you imagine the gentle lapping of the waves? Or the scent of salt water in the air?

We are multisensory beings, so it is quite possible that you will realize that all these senses come into play in your memories and your daydreams. Intuitive impressions may present themselves to your inner awareness through your dominant sense, at least initially. As you open up to receive them more often, they are more likely to come to you with multisensory complexity and depth. Of course, you may also discover that you are one of those people who know something intuitively without knowing how you know.

When you have completed this task, be grateful for whatever new awareness of your abilities these reflections have awarded you. Allow this increased self-knowledge to be subtly, gently transforming. Integrate what you have learned about yourself and become comfortable with it. In doing so, in reacquainting yourself with your inner senses and recognizing your natural proficiency, you will be making a claim to greater healing and empowerment.

3

RECLAIMING THE GIFTS OF THE PAST

One of the ways of becoming more intuitive in the present is to recall the past, exploring memory with the intention of unearthing buried and forgotten moments of intuition and illumination. These memories mark an opening to spiritual guidance and to grace, the conscious awareness of the presence of Spirit. Looking at the past with the intention of recovering these memories is a way to discover the hidden history of the soul. Observing the feelings evoked by these memories also has value: here are clues to present-day confidence or caution regarding the use of intuition.

Isn't that a curious idea—that we each have a hidden history of the soul? We have so many memories, and so many levels and kinds of memory. Yet we are quite capable of selecting specific events to share when we are asked to write a brief biography for a school directory or a business brochure. We are also capable of recalling more revealing details of our lives when we make new friends or want to deepen relationships with old friends. We choose the events of our lives that we will highlight in presenting ourselves to the public. We choose the events that we will share when we want to establish or renew a personal relationship. We also choose, on some level, the events that we allow ourselves to remember and those we prefer to forget—and these choices help us forge a sense of identity.

Memory both reveals and conceals, selecting or foregrounding in our conscious awareness those events that are important to us as turning points and acceptable for presentation. (As an analogy, think of a file drawer in which the files that are used most often are kept in the front.) Other events, which are also significant to us but perhaps not as suitable for sharing, occupy the middle ground of the subconscious. (Think of a second set of files, not so well worn, a bit further back in the same drawer.) Then there are events, which may or may not be significant to us at the time they occur, that we do not want to remember or share, perhaps because the events are painful or confusing, frightening, or inexplicable. The memories of these events are stored in the deep subconscious. (To continue the same analogy, these files are way in the back, their labels not even visible to the eye when you open the drawer.) Memories from infancy and very early childhood that precede the formation of the ego and a separate sense of self, as well as memories of extremely traumatic events, may be stored even more deeply—in the unconscious—so that there is no possibility of remembering them. (These files go directly into underground storage.)

Where do we store the memories of those events that mark turning points in the life of the soul? Clearly, some of our experience is conscious: easily recalled, readily shared. Yet much of it may not be so easily accessed because it occurred in a context in which we felt little or no support for our heightened spiritual awareness. Children who describe invisible friends are sometimes ridiculed or told they'll "grow out of it." Children who see auras are scolded for not coloring inside the lines. Children who describe events from past lives are chided for making up stories. Oft-repeated family histories and images from favorite photo albums tend to reinforce only specific, shared memories, making the truth of individual experience more elusive.

Most of us place a very high value on our connections to our families, our communities, our culture. Because of this, if we meet with initial or ongoing discouragement or opposition from those we love when we attempt to understand our individual spiritual experience, we may learn to avoid it or deny it ourselves.

This repression is a "normal" response, in the sense of it being usual or typical; it enables us to maintain our accepted place within the family and within the larger social systems of the community and culture. This repression can make the task of recalling moments of intuition and illumination more difficult.

For these reasons, engaging in this particular form of self-reflection may seem a lot like panning for gold, sifting through the silt and sediment of the river of time and memory for what shines with soft, glowing brightness. One shake of the pan may not show much. It may be necessary to shake repeatedly, looking again, and then again, to bring those gold nuggets of transcendent individual experiences to light. Do recognize that any that turn up may be crusted with mud and need some washing before they are able to be appreciated for what they are.

REMEMBERING THE PATH TO REIKI

"Let's go around the circle and introduce ourselves to each other. Please tell everyone your name and describe how you first learned about Reiki. Would you like to begin?" I ask, looking at the woman who sits beside me. I smile to encourage her and she begins her story. Eventually, however, the circle returns to me. The length of time this exercise has taken will determine whether I describe my own journey to Reiki quickly or in detail.

If I am concerned about moving on to the next topic of discussion, I will say that ever since I was a child I have been interested in healing. My mother had seven miscarriages before I was six years old, so I was aware, at a very young age, of how much I wanted to be able to do something to relieve the suffering of those I love. This interest in healing remained with me throughout my schooling. I was even a pre-med major in my freshman year of college, until I blanked out on a final chemistry exam and had to admit to myself that I wasn't a good candidate for such a competitive career. Years later, when I learned about Reiki, it seemed like an answer to a prayer.

End of story.

However, if time allows, I will mention this event. One Saturday afternoon in late September of my second year of graduate studies in English at Temple University, I wanted a break from my books and so I decided to go to a holistic fair on the grounds of nearby Rosemont College. I meandered through the booths and displays until I finally settled into a a lecture on Native American medicine. Much of what the speaker said was already familiar to me, yet I stayed. Finally the speaker invited questions from the audience. A pleasant-looking woman asked such an insightful question that I decided I wanted to meet her. After the lecture concluded I moved through the crowd to where she stood and introduced myself. In turn, she told me her name and explained that she did shamanic journeying and Reiki.

"Reiki. I want to learn that," I said, startling myself.

"Do you know what it is?" she asked, looking perplexed.

I smiled and shook my head. "No, I have no idea. I just know that I want to learn it. What is it?"

She took this in stride and began to explain: "It's a form of hands-on healing, but it is hard to describe. You really need to experience it to understand it. You should come for a treatment." She gave me her number, and I decided to make an appointment for a treatment in her Chestnut Hill office.

Three weeks later, as I lay on her bodywork table asking questions and listening carefully to her answers, my impressions, and the flow of energy through her hands, I was still resolute. "I want to learn this," I told her. "Where can I find a teacher?"

"You just missed Beth Gray. She'll be back in the area again next spring—in about six months. You'll have to wait."

That was in the fall of 1986. When Reverend Beth Gray returned to Bucks County on her next visit in March 1987, she taught Reiki in a private home to a handful of students, and I was one of them.

LOOKING DEEPER

Usually, after sharing this story with my students, I simply move on to describe the nature of Reiki healing. Sometimes, however, I share the lessons that I took away from that experience and have only understood later, upon reflection. Like many people who are guided to Reiki I knew, without knowing how I knew, that I was meant to learn it—and I knew this without having any understanding of what Reiki is.

Although I had to wait six months to take a class, I was completely committed to doing so. Yet during the class, which I attended over three days, I fidgeted in my seat as I listened to Beth Gray's lectures. Though I felt I was supposed to be there, I also felt skeptical; and I nearly bolted from my chair during the first of the four traditional attunements, because I was unprepared for any ritual that had me putting my hands in prayer position. At the end of the class I thought my hands felt different, charged and energized, but I thought a thousand other things as well. My mind reeled trying to make sense of all that I had heard and experienced. I felt divided and confused.

Not surprisingly, I was not sure how to introduce Reiki into my life. By practicing hand positions on myself as I lay in bed, drifting off to sleep or slowly awakening on a leisurely Saturday morning, I learned through my own experience that Reiki relaxes and calms and clarifies the senses. And, just as Beth Gray had predicted, as I listened to my hands I learned to notice more and more subtle changes in the flow of healing energy. However, I felt no great courage to take Reiki anywhere beyond my own closed doors, for I had no confidence in its ability to relax or bring healing to anyone else.

I had followed my guidance, but I had followed it blindly: I had learned Reiki, but the class had not revealed enough to me to clearly understand it or explain it to anyone else. I was caught up in a mystery—and I was to remain so for some time to come, until I was invited to treat my first client, a lame horse named Holly, whom my Reiki Master, Beth Gray, would later call my first Reiki miracle.* Not until Holly recovered completely did I offer to do Reiki hands-on healing on anyone else.

This sequence of events is not uncommon: we are guided in the direction of our own highest good and greatest spiritual growth, which may or may not be

---

*For more about the Reiki treatments on Holly, see my book *Traditional Reiki for Our Times*, pp. 22–23.

marked by a moment of transformation, but our growth usually comes gently and gradually, through experience over time. When we learn Reiki, we are granted a moment of transformation with each attunement. Like a fertile seed planted in rich soil, the energy of the attunement grows and pushes upward into our lives. Through our practice, it is nurtured to fruition. We feel it as a blossoming of love in our hearts, in our minds, in our souls.

Now, many years later, I understand that Reiki is the teacher, and the lessons it teaches continue long after the official close of class. I can see that I was given both guidance and the opportunity to grow and heal spiritually through my experience of Reiki. Yet in retrospect it still seems odd that I could be, at one and the same time, so wisely guided to Reiki and so resistant and slow to recognize its value.

This conundrum offers some clues to the workings of Reiki and intuition: if we are open to being guided, we will be guided; if we close down or resist, we may miss the opportunities guidance presents. Yet ultimately, if we persist in our spiritual practice, we will heal enough to become open again and to appreciate our experience.

AND LOOKING DEEPER STILL

There is, of course, another question that occurred to me after additional reflection. What possessed me to blurt out those words to the woman I met at the lecture? Why was I so willing to be guided? How did I know, on any level, that I wanted to learn Reiki, when I had never heard of it before?

To answer that question I had to remind myself of a whole series of decisions that I had made three years earlier: I would be patient with the process of healing. I would let myself feel and grieve. I would allow myself to be creative in familiar and new ways. I would reevaluate old interests and discover some new ones. I would keep a dream diary. I would learn more about my intuition and develop it into a source of guidance that I could trust.

These decisions came out of a determination to rebuild myself and my life after two devastating losses drove me into severe depression. The year was 1983. Between the snows of early February and the flowers of late March, I lost both the man and the work I loved. I felt devastated. I thought again and again about taking a curve too fast on a country road and driving into a tree. I imagined the twisted wreckage, the sirens. What stopped me was synchronicity, two extraordinary coincidences that I could not easily dismiss.

One afternoon I came home to find an after-school special called *Amy's Angel* playing on the TV. This modern retelling of *It's a Wonderful Life* showed a would-be angel who had to earn his wings by preventing the suicide of a depressed teenage girl named Amy. I plunked down on the couch, kicked off my shoes, and watched. Here, was a story—with my name on it—that compelled me to think again about the worth of my life and the impact of the suicide I contemplated on the people I loved. I determined I would try to endure, even though I was constantly aware of my own terrible sadness.

The fight against depression was not easy. I still had suicidal thoughts, although now I rejected them and deliberately turned my attention to something else. Over time I began to claim moments, then hours, in which I was at least distracted from the emotional pain, if not depression-free. I began to take better care of myself, despite the indifference to life that I still felt.

One night in April 1983 I decided to go upstairs to my room at about 9:30 PM and to dress for bed in the dark. For some reason I simply wanted to sit by my window and watch the night sky. For several minutes I admired it—a peaceful spring night sky, a cool, soft breeze, twinkling stars.

And then the light in the sky to the west and overhead began to get brighter and glow softly red. I thought about a fire in the fields and woods below, or even at the neighbor's house in the valley, but there was no crackling sound and no smoke—only a soft, reddening glow. My mind began to reach for more extreme possibilities: a police car's flashing lights, the red glare of a gun battle, a UFO. My heart pounded. All of these possibilities alarmed me, but none seemed to fit. The fields and woods below me were quiet and peaceful, in marked contrast to the drama being played out above.

I scanned the night sky again and watched, astonished, as emerald green ribbons of light unfurled from an unseen point overhead. They "settled" in the northeast quadrant of the sky, where they shimmered and undulated against the red glow that now completely veiled the darkness.

Only then did I realize what I saw: the northern lights, aurora borealis, on an April night, far to the south of the Arctic Circle and the Canadian border, almost as far south as the Mason-Dixon line, and far beyond the geography of my imagination.

I put a down coat over my nightgown, donned my slippers, and went outside. I lay on my back on the cold ground, staring upward at the heavens, and watched the dance of light to a celestial music that I could not hear, but with which I felt in harmony.

I understood, at last, that this particular display of God's own fireworks was one I was meant to see. I had listened to that gentle prompting to go upstairs to bed early, to sit by the window in the darkness, to look at the night sky. Where had that impulse come from? My intuition? My guardian angel? God? Whatever its source, by attending to it I came to realize that I am guided and loved by a higher power—as we all are—and in that understanding I took comfort and received healing.

The message of the northern lights enabled me to have faith that I would heal from the two losses I had endured. Learning how to heal was *hard* spiritual work—and this work transformed me. I searched for and found humor. I struggled to understand and to forgive. I decided to take a few deliberate risks in order to create opportunities for good in my life. I moved to the suburbs of Washington, D.C., where I found work doing marketing for an architectural firm. I deliberately revisited a couple of childhood ambitions for another look: besides being a writer and besides being a doctor or healer of some sort, I had wanted to be an astronaut, so I took a course in engineering calculus at a community college in Virginia and began taking flying lessons. Short of soloing, I stopped, at least certain that I could still be inspired into awe by the colors of the sunrise.

After about a year and a half of avoiding writing and shutting out my dreams, I realized that I missed them both. I asked Spirit to help me to write and prayed to dream again. A wonderful book entitled *Creative Dreaming,* by Patricia Garfield, inspired me to try to remember my dreams again by recording whatever fragments I recalled on waking in a dream journal. Soon I began to write in this journal daily. I recognized that my dreams were a source of healing, the practice of recording them a healing meditation.

During the following year I returned to Pennsylvania to begin graduate studies at Temple University. While I was busy during the day with classes and reading assignments, I still found time to think more about the role of intuition in my life. Though it had been on and off again throughout my childhood and young adulthood, listening to it had saved my life. I realized that Spirit was willing to work with me—to open me up or close me off to my intuition, as I asked. So I asked to be opened up again, not only to receive warning messages, but also to receive guidance that was positive or neutral in its emotional charge. If I was to feel the responsibility, at times, of being a messenger, then I also wanted to feel some lightness and joy in allowing myself to be guided by Spirit.

This prayer was quickly answered with a vivid dream in which I saw a string of bright red chili peppers. The next day I shared an unexpected and very pleasant lunch with a graduate school friend. Hanging above our booth, behind his head, were those red chili peppers. Since I was now keeping a dream journal, I noted both the dream and its validation—and allowed myself to open up more to my intuition.

As a result, on that day a year later, when I first heard the name Reiki at Rosemont College's Holistic Health Fair, I was only a little surprised to hear myself say, "I want to learn that!" More important, I knew that I was being guided, and that I must honor that guidance by taking a Reiki class as soon as one was available.

DISCOVERING MORE OF THE HIDDEN HISTORY OF THE SOUL

Did you notice how briefly I mentioned my on-and-off-again experiences with intuition in childhood and young adulthood? Many people dismiss their earliest experiences of intuition and awareness of the sacred. These experiences don't fit into the accepted forms of life-story telling: resume, bio, profile, memoir. Yet every single human being could tell just such a story, given enough time for reflection and the courage to face the past. Yes, it does take courage to remember experiences with intuition that may have seemed confusing or frightening, if not initially, then in retrospect.

When I acknowledged to myself that there might be a value in looking across the length of my lifetime to find moments of intuition and illumination, I felt daunted by the task. Fortunately, I didn't think of myself as a particularly intuitive person, so I didn't expect to find a lot of them! I soon realized that in order to fully reclaim my intuition, I needed to identify not only the moments when I had been aware of my inner guidance, but also my response to that awareness. Did I feel pleased to have a tiny glimpse of the future? Was I frightened by what I saw? Did I feel comfortable sharing my intuitive impressions with others? Did I mind being thought of as different?

At the end of this chapter I will invite you to undertake this review of long-ago memories and to consider these same questions. You may choose to look back from the present to the past, to begin with your first memory and work forward, or to enter the past through any one of the many doors along the way—those significant events, such as a move cross country, the start of a new job, the birth of a child, that mark turning points in your own life. You may also sift through memory for experiences of particular kinds of intuition: inner seeing, hearing, smell, and so on. When you finish this review you will have a deeper understanding of the ways in which intuition works for you, the obstacles you or those around you raised against it, and the support you were given for it.

My own review revealed several precognitive dreams and a few early experiences of knowing without knowing how I knew. My family taught me to value my dreams, but I resisted describing to anyone the instances of uncanny knowledge, tamping down the physical sensations that accompanied them. In doing so, I denied myself the possibility of support from family or friends. Here are a few examples of my finds.

When I was about nine years old I had a pleasant dream that I remembered on waking: I saw myself packing a suitcase because I had been invited to stay for a week with my favorite cousins, even though I did not own a suitcase and I had never stayed with them before. I said nothing to anyone in my family about the dream but I remembered it throughout the day, holding it close because it was pleasant and comforting to think about. To my astonishment and delight, the next day I overheard my mother talking on the phone to my Aunt Margie. I could tell that they were discussing the possibility of me visiting my cousins. Without any prompting from me, my mother and my aunt were giving me my dream come true, by together deciding that my summer vacation should include this special visit.

This was something I pondered on the hour-long car drive as I sat quietly in the backseat, beside the borrowed suitcase packed with my clothes and a few precious belongings. How had my mother and my aunt known that I would love to visit my cousins when I hadn't said a word? Had they ever talked about this before? Had my dream somehow delivered a message to them? Or had this trip simply been arranged in advance, on some other level of love, before any words were spoken about it?

My sense of what was possible in this world, on this planet, subtly changed. Unfortunately, this dream—telling me in advance of something wonderful on the way—was a singular event during my childhood. However, my parents, both artists, by their own example encouraged me to value my dreams. Each morning, as they drank their coffee, my father would tell my mother and my brother and me about his dreams, which were often complete stories. Once in a while my mother would describe one of her dreams, usually of a painting she would like to do or a clay sculpture she wanted to build. While this encouragement to value dreams may seem insignificant, it was not: creativity and dreams draw from the same deep well of the individual and collective unconscious; intuition taps this well for the water of hidden feeling and brings it up to the light of awareness for healing, release, and joy. Only in retrospect have I come to understand that by teaching me to value dreams, creativity, and intuition, my parents gave me a great inheritance.

My mother offered me the greatest support. Still thinking about my dream and wondering at the ease with which we all understood my Italian-speaking grandmother, I asked my mother questions about how people can communicate without words. She told me that when people love or care for one other, sometimes they share a bond that allows them to know when they are needed. The example she gave me was a personal one: she and her sister had discovered that sometimes when one of them telephoned the other, the line would be busy—and later they would laugh together about it, because they realized that they had been trying to call each other at the same time.

My mother, who was of Irish-Italian ancestry, told me that the Irish believed in something called second sight—a way of seeing or knowing events at a distance without being physically present. The seer might observe events that happened lifetimes ago, or that were yet to happen, or that were occurring now but miles away, far beyond the range of our physical eyesight.

She told me she herself had been fascinated by the story of Bridey Murphy, a young woman who, under hypnosis, recalled details of a past life that were later verified by a researcher; she had also read some of Edgar Cayce's writing, and she particularly enjoyed science fiction that addressed this issue of communication without words. She put into my hands anthologies that included John Wyndham's "Rebirth" and John Varley's "Peripheral Vision"; she lent me her paperback edition of Zenna Henderson's *People*. Here was wonder: telepaths who could not only read one another's thoughts while in the same room, but who could talk, mind to mind, to one another across a distance of many miles. In this way, my mother encouraged me to learn more and to reflect upon my own rare experiences with intuition.

About ten years after that first precognitive dream, during the summer between my junior and senior year of college, I had major surgery. During the six-week recovery period following the operation, I found myself having disquieting dreams: I dreamt that I was awake, with my hand on the knob of my bedroom door, trying to turn the knob. Then I would awaken and realize that I was not standing at the door at all. I was still in bed, with my arm flung above my head on the pillow. Or I would dream that I was awake, turning on the light by the door. As hard as I tried to flick the switch, I could not do it. Again, I would awake to find myself still in bed, with my hand resting on the pillow beside my face. These dreams happened over and over, and I found them frightening because I could not tell what was real and what was not.

A college friend, who had just graduated with a major in anthropology, asked me if I might be astral projecting. The idea was outlandish to me. How could I? She said that sometimes when people have surgery their sense of connection to the physical body changes and they become freer to move around in their sleep state. I found this terrifying, just as I had found the dreams. Some people cultivated the ability to travel out-of-body, she told me. Although I was relieved to know what I was doing, I did not enjoy the experience. I hated the lack of control and the inability to tell what was real. I prayed that such dreams would end, and eventually they did.

Almost a decade later, during the years I worked at a publishing company in rural Pennsylvania, I dreamed of a coworker who had been diagnosed with breast cancer who had left the company shortly after I arrived to live with one of her sisters in the Midwest. In the dream she was in a queue for an outdoor shower that shimmered with water and light. She was afraid. Somehow, when I woke from the dream, I knew that she had very little time to live. I didn't like dreaming a dream foretelling death; I wasn't happy to be the bearer of bad news. But despite my reservations, I shared the dream with two of this woman's closest friends in Pennsylvania and encouraged them to get in touch with her. When she died soon after, I comforted myself with the knowledge that they had been able to say good-bye.

Sometime later I experienced another out-of-body dream, only in this dream I felt much more comfortable. I traveled through the wall of my bedroom, through the wooden framing and insulation of the walls of the house, and floated in the sky admiring the bright moon above the woods. I could see the silver cord that trailed behind me back to my body, and I did not feel afraid. As soon as I thought of returning to my body, I was back in an instant.

Because I wanted to remember more of my dreams, I later decided to keep a dream journal. Not every dream was meaningful, but by recording whatever I remembered on waking I came to appreciate the variety and power of dreams. As my appreciation increased, so did the frequency of significant dreams. I learned through experience that dreams are an avenue of connection between the subconscious and the conscious mind, and between inner wisdom and ordinary awareness; I came to understand how well dreams can serve to heal, inspire, and guide us.

Besides dreams, the other way that I received information intuitively was to know, without knowing how I knew. Sometimes this knowing was accompanied by a tangle of knots in my belly or a feeling of intense anxiety, a presentiment of danger or disaster. The first time this occurred, at thirteen, I was unable to dismiss the foreboding that I felt day after day in regard to a particular friend, until the morning I was told that he had been charged with a crime. The next time this occurred I was twenty: I found myself in a department store at a scarf counter, holding two black scarves, confounded by the certainty that someone I knew was going to die. When I was told later that day that a friend had threatened suicide, I asked my husband to call 911 and an ambulance, which helped to save my friend's life.

These experiences made me recall a childhood trip to Roadside America, a tourist attraction featuring an enormous model railroad display. A miniature panorama of an entire city had stretched out before me. Trains moved. Signals blinked on and off. What really caught my attention, though, was a flicker of flames from a burning building in the middle of the panorama.

It was upsetting to think that my intuition might work only by registering those future events with a high negative emotional charge. This is one reason that I resisted "owning" the gift of intuition.

Of course, I was glad and grateful to help prevent a suicide, but why hadn't I been able to help my other friend when he had gotten into trouble? My intuition, if I had it at all, seemed to be hit or miss. How could I trust it when it operated so rarely? How could I know when I was right and when I was wrong? When I received a message in this way, what was my responsibility? Overwhelmed by such questions, I decided that I wasn't really sure that I wanted to be intuitive at all. Without a commitment on my part to claim my intuition, I shut down—not all the way, but part of the way. This slowed my progress in accepting intuition as my inner connection to Spirit.

Another experience of knowing without knowing how occurred roughly ten years later, in my late twenties. One morning I woke up with knots in my stomach, a sense of dread, and a particular friend on my mind. What was going on with him? I waited until noon to make the long-distance call from my office to ask. He told me that he and a friend had been talking about going out that night to look for a good bar fight. He knew enough bars in Boston to find one, he felt sure. "Please don't do this," I begged. I explained the strange foreboding that had wakened me that morning and eventually persuaded him to find a tamer form of entertainment for the evening. Once I had his reassurance, the tangle of knots in my stomach relaxed and I was able to breathe more easily.

The next events of any significance in my (soul's) life story are those two disastrous losses which I have already described. Although they took away from me both love and work, they gave me experiences that taught me, at last, to appreciate and honor my intuition. I continue to learn about intuition, as I use it with Reiki as a tool for healing and guidance. I now recognize intuition is a gift from Spirit which enables me to know that I am connected to universal life-force energy in another way; sensing the subtle energy of impressions as Reiki flows into me, through my crown and past my third eye and my throat and my heart, is simply an expansion of the ability to sense the subtle energy of Reiki as it moves on, and flows into and through my hands to bring healing.

SUGGESTIONS FOR PRACTITIONERS

Do you remember digging for buried treasure when you were a child? Do you recall how excited you were to be pushing aside the soil with your fingers in the hope—and positive expectancy—that you would find something worthwhile? A real arrowhead, perhaps? A piece of broken pottery from early settlers? Gold coins forgotten by a leprechaun or fairies? Do you remember how your feelings shifted toward disappointment and resigned acceptance when all you found was a squirrel's buried nut, a bird's feather, a few dirty pennies?

If you were a fortunate child, someone pointed out to you that the nut was the squirrel's hidden treasure, a secret stash of food for the winter—and the seed of a tree as well. The feather, however ordinary it might seem, could be used to make a quill pen or to perform a Native American ceremony; with help, you could learn how to shape the quill into a nib and try it out yourself as a writing instrument, or you might ornament it with leather and beads and shells and transform it into a smudge wand. Those old pennies might simply have fallen out of the pocket of a passerby and might not be worth much, but they did have a value and could make a difference between being able to buy popcorn at the movies or not.

Approach the task of reflecting on your own life with the enthusiasm and excitement of a child searching for buried treasure. Be patient. Be willing to be amazed by what you find, however ordinary it might seem. Be willing to look at it again and again, considering the practical purpose it served in your life at the time and the spiritual purpose it served then and may still be serving now. Notice the feelings the memory evokes. If you notice shock, surprise, embarrassment, self-doubt, or fear, see who else is peopling the landscape of your memory. You may be recalling first the emotional response of your parents or peers, allowing it to filter out the purity of your own experience; or you may be rejecting the experience out of cultural conditioning. Keep scraping away the layers of remembered feelings associated with the event until you arrive at a clearer idea of the facts and your own response to those facts, before any other person had offered comment or criticism.

NOW YOU

The self-appointed task of reflecting on memories is much like sitting beside a moving stream. It requires that you relax and become quiet, to still yourself, in order to see beyond the dazzle of favorite memories of shared times and familiar turning-point events. In your safe place, let yourself relax and become centered and quiet. Then let yourself remember. Work with the intention of discovering the days that will disclose to you the hidden history of your soul. These are, at once, more ordinary *and* extraordinary than other days of your life. Because of this, recalling them may take more effort.

Whether you approach this task of remembrance as meditation or journaling, ease yourself into it by deciding to identify a specific, single thread of experience over the length of your lifetime. For example, what was your earliest spiritual experience? How did you feel? Did you keep your experience to yourself or did you share it with someone? Did this person make you feel supported or discouraged? What was your spiritual life like in your teens? Did you find yourself feeling alone or were you comforted by a sense of community? Did these feelings change as you entered your twenties and began to live more independently? Do you distinguish your religious life from your spiritual life, or are they inseparable? Do you have a sense of yourself, over the course of your life, as an evolving soul? What experiences have nurtured you? What has confused you or made you falter on your spiritual path? What has gotten you back "on course"? You might, in later sessions, look at other threads of experience: dreams, deja vu, knowings, and so on.

Another way to engage in this archaeology of the soul is to look back at your life more broadly, but across a much shorter period of time, and then to repeat the process looking at another time period. For example, during the last five years have you had any dreams that seemed to offer guidance? Have you allowed yourself to make any important decisions by following a hunch or because "it just felt right"? Have you visited a psychic or a tarot card reader? Did you feel any of the information presented to you was of value, or did you quickly dismiss it because of someone else's ridicule?

This task is, essentially, a life review. Please don't expect to accomplish the work of recollection and reevaluation in one sitting. Be patient. Whether you work with one thread of experience or several threads, whether you review a short or a long period of time, be willing to give this task your relaxed attention and loving care. Be willing to repeat it as often as necessary until you feel you have taken a thorough look at the hidden history of your soul and have a good understanding of your own intuitive nature and preferences. (This life review can also be accomplished through guided visualization, or, for those who enjoy hypnotherapy, through multiple regressions.)

Your purpose in undertaking this life review is to identify those intuitive gifts with which you were born and those that you developed in childhood, adolescence, and young adulthood, so that you may reclaim those abilities at the Reiki table as a practitioner. Your path to Reiki is likely to offer you valuable clues. If you can identify not only the obvious connections that brought you to Reiki, but the turning points in your spiritual path that led you here, you are likely to gain a very different view of your own history than you have ever had before.

Your decision to learn Reiki is, very likely, the culmination of a long series of events, some challenging and some inspiring, that were significant to you as a soul. If you can identify those events, your reaction to those events, and the influence on you of the reactions of others, you will gain a liberating sense of perspective and an appreciation for yourself as a spiritual being that you may never have had before.

☙

Those who read the Bible will be familiar with these words, recorded in the Gospel of Matthew 7:7: "Ask, and it shall be given; seek, and ye shall find; knock, and it shall be opened unto you." Once you have completed your life review you may realize that, on one or more occasions, you have shut down, closed off, or denied spiritual or intuitive experience. You may even have prayed to God to end the disconcerting dreams, visions, or knowings. If you have done so, take a closer look at these particular experiences and the reasons they have aroused such fear.

Is it time now to ask that the door to a particular kind of spiritual or intuitive experience may again be open to you? I do not think that I will ever pray to be able to see ghosts, although I recognize that there is a place for this spiritual ability. However, I am glad that I prayed that I might be able to dream again. My dreams remain a source of healing, beauty, wonder, creativity, inspiration, and guidance.

Ask Spirit to return to you any spiritual or intuitive gifts that you denied or refused that you now would like to reclaim. Be grateful that this request is already granted. Continue your prayer as long as feels necessary or appropriate. Know that you will be able to reclaim this gift at the perfect time, or you will come to the awareness that this is one gift you no longer need. If so, just let go. Know that there will be other gifts of Spirit for you along the way.

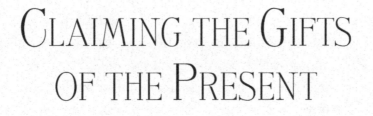

CLAIMING THE GIFTS
OF THE PRESENT

"'Intuitive development is spiritual development.'"

Linda Schiller-Hanna, a professional psychic and trainer, spoke in a firm, authoritative voice that was amplified electronically so that even the members of the audience crowded into the back of the huge conference room could hear her. She and co-presenter Mary Roach, also a professional psychic with an international clientele, were leading a workshop on intuitive development for the Association for Research and Enlightenment, founded by Edgar Cayce in the early 1930s. "This is something that Edgar Cayce himself said when people challenged the validity of his work: 'intuitive development is spiritual development,'" Schiller-Hanna said again.

I sat in the audience, quietly listening, inwardly reeling from the impact of this simple statement. With just a few of Cayce's words, now shared in this workshop, the last of my doubts and fears about the nature and source of intuition had been laid to rest, and an important connection had been made. To grow intuitively would be to grow spiritually. To commit to developing my intuition would be to step forward with more determination on my spiritual path. To work on advancing my intuition, without attachment to results, would be equivalent in some ways to practicing meditation without engaging in any struggle with my thoughts.

A Reiki friend and member of the Association for Research and Enlightenment (A.R.E.) had invited me to attend this workshop as one of her guests, and I had accepted her invitation with anticipation. After taking Reiki II with Beth Gray in 1987 and experiencing my own on-again, off-again ability to receive intuitive impressions while doing Reiki, I had come to understand that I wanted to learn all that I could about intuition and my own intuitive ability so that I could be as accurate as possible in presenting impressions to my clients and as responsible and appropriate as any professional reader.

I had been reading several books about intuition and psychic development. I had listened intently to Sonia Choquette's book *Your Psychic Pathway* on tape and had attempted to apply the principles and practice some of the exercises. I had wished for the opportunity to practice with others in a workshop setting, and now here I was: at an A.R.E. workshop on intuitive development as a member's guest. This, I recognized, was a synchronicity—a happy "coincidence"—that matched reality to my desire and a gift from Spirit offered in the present. What could I do but say yes?

The workshop proved to be important in many ways. It deepened my understanding of the nature of intuition; it demonstrated, through practice sessions with partners, that intuition is an ability we all possess; it gave me some guidelines for appropriate methods of presentation; and it allowed me to experience the healing that an intuitive impression, shared with gentleness and compassion, can initiate.

Athough I took this workshop in April 1999, I still take advantage of any opportunities that are presented to me to learn more about intuition, because intuition is enhanced by Reiki, because it enhances Reiki treatments, and because I find this a fascinating subject to study. Workshops, books, training tapes and CDs are all "gifts of the present" that we can use to gain confidence and comfort with our intuition and with intuitive Reiki. (For a list of recommended workshops, see Appendix 2; for a list of recommended books, see Suggested Reading.)

Yet there are some gifts that we can claim that require no application or order form and that cost nothing. The most fundamental is life itself—and life experience. We can reflect on our life experience using our intelligence; we can recall the past through memory; we can envision the future and create it through imagination.

Beyond that, we can use our free will to choose to learn skills and develop areas of expertise. By using the ability to read and to comprehend written and spoken language you may claim access to many other kinds of knowledge, from survival skills in the wilderness (how to light a fire, build a shelter, forage for food) to success skills in the workplace (how to write a resume, present yourself at a job interview, manage time). You may also choose to explore, through reading or lectures, esoteric or mystical knowledge (the power of prayer, the possibility of reincarnation, the philosophy of Buddhism).

If you are willing and able to engage your physical body, as well as your mind, in the learning process, you may acquire many more skills of personal and practical value. (How to paint a watercolor, throw clay on a potter's wheel, play the French horn, raft down a river, lasso a calf, sail by the stars, perform tai chi, practice yoga, learn Reiki—the list of possibilities goes on.)

Truly, knowledge is power, and the free will choices that we make to learn skills and gain expertise in certain areas of knowledge help to define us. Yet there is another free will choice that may have an even more profound effect on the quality of life: attitude. Viktor E. Frankl, in his book *Man's Search for Meaning,* describes the harsh conditions, the terrible awareness of loss, and the constant threat of death he and his fellow prisoners endured in the Nazi concentration camps of World War II. In seeking to understand why and how he and some of his fellow prisoners survived when so many millions died, he acknowledges the power of attitude. By freely choosing positive thoughts, beliefs, and expectations over negative thoughts, cynicism, and despair, he believes we increase our chances of survival and, more important, of spiritual growth.

Will we reach for light, for illumination of the meaning and purpose of our lives and the sense of empowerment, peace of mind, and joy that accompanies that knowledge? Or will we allow ourselves to dwell in darkness, unwilling to release the hold of a difficult past or drawn down into a mire of negativity by some present circumstance? Whether we choose a positive or a negative attitude, our choice will affect us deeply, body and mind, heart and soul.

Fortunately, the present moment holds the greatest possibility. It is never too soon and never too late to begin to live with awareness, intention, and gratitude. Like other spiritual practices, choosing to approach life with a positive attitude is not a once-and-done accomplishment. It is a discipline, a deliberate choice we make again and again and again, sometimes with ease and sometimes only with determined effort.

Gradually this spiritual discipline enables us to see our lives in a steady, positive light, despite appearances to the contrary; and eventually those appearances alter to fit our positive attitude: our life-affirming thoughts, beliefs, and expectations. (Affirmations derive their power from this metaphysical principle, which is acknowledged in our culture by sayings such as "mind over matter," "seeing is believing," and "you create your own reality.")

Many of us take the gifts of life, consciousness, and free will for granted. Yet these are the foundation of being and becoming who we are and who we are meant to be: they enable us to define our identities, to develop moral character and values, and to claim spiritual growth. In practicing Reiki and in meditating on the Reiki principles, it is good to remember these gifts, common to us all, and to be grateful for them.

Our families and our cultures also influence our development as individuals, offering us a context for understanding our life experiences and ourselves. We may assimilate the values these social systems present without question; we may accept them with or without reservations; or we may reject some as unworthy or unworkable. Though we may count our family life as a great blessing, our religious traditions as sacred, our country's heritage as proud, we can do so only because we are alive, conscious, and possessed of free will. These are the first and most fundamental gifts of the present.

THE GIFT OF REIKI

Sometimes when I am asked about Reiki I say that choosing to learn Reiki was the best decision I have made in my adult life. The ability to bring healing to those I love and to myself through this simple, natural method is soul-satisfying, and the impact of witnessing profound healing has been transforming. As I have witnessed more and more "miracles" my doubt and skepticism have dissolved and been replaced by faith, and my faith has been tempered through the fire of experience into knowledge. Like a strong sword, it has a heft and weight to it. It can be used with gentle force to carve away another's doubts and to clear the way for courage and hope and the possibility of healing. This is one of the benefits of years of Reiki experience.

Yet Reiki offers it practitioners many other blessings, which may be more quickly received. Whether we do Reiki on a client or on ourselves, we always receive some healing. We may feel calmer and more relaxed, gain clarity, or simply feel a sense of greater well-being. These are immediate effects. With consistent Reiki practice, they become enduring. Eventually we recognize that we have been healed in more ways than we ever imagined possible.

When we do Reiki, we do not do healing. Instead, we serve as channels for the healing force of universal life-force energy, which is transferred primarily through our hands. Though this is a passive role, we may take pleasure and pride in our willingness to actively serve in this role and to do so with integrity and kindness. By acknowledging ourselves in this way, we begin to claim our empowerment.

Committed Reiki practice brings profound healing to practitioners and clients and creates positive changes in relationships, in communities, and in the world. When we say "yes" to the daily discipline of self-treatment and to any opportunities to do Reiki as service that come our way, we are gently claiming our own eventual enlightenment and inviting enlightenment—an increase in light, well-being, and wisdom—around the globe.

REIKI HANDS

Once we are attuned as Reiki practitioners, our hands grasp the rope that has been tossed down to us from above, and we begin to climb to the heavens! Of course, this is not literally true. Instead, we use our hands—large or small, white or black or yellow or red, rough and coarsened or refined and polished—in service. We treat ourselves to Reiki each day. We treat a sister, a brother, a father, a friend, a fellow athlete, a coworker or colleague, and an occasional stranger. As a result, we experience healing and we bring healing to others that slowly, gently has a positive impact on our immediate world.

Now multiply that action by the millions of Reiki practitioners in the world (a number which increases daily). Imagine how the impact of each practitioner's efforts ripples out, reinforcing the efforts of other practitioners. See how the world is transformed and remapped by Reiki light?

So we are transformed as well into beings of light, whose hands are charged with a healing energy that is perceptible to us as practitioners and to our clients. The soothing warmth, the cooling comfort, the tingling, the pulsing, the swirling of energy vortices under a palm or a fingertip are all perceptions of the subtle energy of Reiki that help us to understand that the energy is flowing and allow us to monitor the flow and to notice when the energy shifts in intensity so that we can move on to the next position.

Traditionally taught Reiki practitioners will be completely familiar with the practice of "listening" to the energy that I have just described. No matter the lineage, no matter whether the practitioner is taught in the Usui Shiki Ryoho tradition (tracing back through Hawayo Takata and Chujiro Hayashi to Mikao Usui), common throughout the world, or the Usui Reiki Ryoho tradition, common in Japan, most of us are taught to make the decision to move our hands from one position to the next by noticing changes in the flow of Reiki energy. (To learn more about the Japanese technique of listening to the energy in the hands, noticing *hibiki,* or "resonance," read chapter 13.)

Listening to the Reiki energy flowing through one's hands is the perfect way to learn how to listen to intuition. The information that is communicated in an intuitive impression floats on the same stream of universal life-force energy that enters us and moves through us to bring healing to our clients and to ourselves. When we have practiced Reiki for a period of time we can feel the pathway of this energy: most often it enters us through the crown and moves down into our hearts, touches us with unconditional love, and then radiates outward, spreading down our arms into our hands, where it is transferred through our hands for the purpose of healing. Occasionally, if the client or the practitioner needs some grounding, we will feel the energy rising up through our feet and legs to blend with the energy from above. Of course, this process may take just a few seconds or several minutes, so we need to be paying close attention to feel it fully.

When we place our hands in position to do Reiki, we place ourselves in what is virtually a shimmering column of light and healing energy. We know this to be universal life-force energy, which brings healing and gentle transformation not only to our clients but to us as well. Over time, we come to recognize that this energy is indeed soul-guided or Spirit-guided. It comes from Source, which creates and sustains life in all its forms, and which heals with an intelligence and wisdom far greater than our own. When we stand within that column of universal life-force energy we are connected to Source, to All-That-Is (a Native American term for Spirit), including all people, all places, all periods of time.

As we do Reiki, Spirit may present information to us, coalescing it out of the light that we watch with the inner eye as the energy streams through us, or presenting it to us to register with another inner sense. What we notice in our hands is one kind of perception of this energy; what we notice with the third eye or the inner ear is simply another kind of perception of the same energy.

This makes learning to receive intuitive impressions an almost inevitable consequence of learning Reiki and committing to Reiki practice, no matter how we are taught. If we are taught traditionally, with repeated attunements and an emphasis on the importance of learning to listen to our hands, then we can look forward to receiving intuitive impressions as we do Reiki in a relatively short period of time. If we are not taught traditionally, with only one attunement and instructions to place our hands in position for so many minutes on the clock, we may wait a bit longer, but over the course of time we will eventually open to receive the inner guidance we seek.

ATTUNEMENTS

As Reiki practitioners, we are privileged to receive attunements which enable us to become channels of universal life-force energy. Whether a practitioner perceives an attunement as gentle and quietly meditative or dramatic and intense does not matter. A Reiki attunement initiates a transformation in conscious awareness and subtle energy perception that continues to develop through Reiki practice, becoming stronger, clearer, deeper, more refined.

Occasionally Reiki Masters offer the practitioners they have trained the opportunity to be reattuned as they assist at a class or at a Reikishare. Sometimes practitioners recognize on their own that an additional attunement would be helpful. Faced with difficult circumstances, a health problem, or severe emotional stress, the practitioner may feel the need for Reiki support. Honor this inner wisdom. Take advantage of the opportunity to be reattuned. Attunements, besides bringing transformation, bring healing, enlightenment, empowerment.

THE REIKI PRINCIPLES

Although the Reiki principles are less emphasized in the West than in Japan, where Mikao Usui's practice of reciting them in his morning and evening meditations is well-known and followed by many practitioners, they deserve consideration and contemplation. Even acquainting yourself with the differences in the presentation of the principles in the West and in Japan has value.

Here is a translation of the original Usui precepts, based on a copy given by Mrs. Kimiko Koyama (chairperson of the Gakkai until January 1998, when Mr. Masayoshi Kondoh assumed the position) to Mr. Hiroshi Doi, a Japanese Reiki Master who has served as an emissary to the West, sharing knowledge of traditional Japanese Reiki techniques.*

The Secret Method to Invite Happiness

THE MIRACLE MEDICINE FOR ALL DISEASES

For today only, do not be angry.
Do not be anxious, and be grateful.

---

*From "Usui Reiki Hikkei—Some Comments," in the *Usui Reiki Ryoho: Shoden, Okuden and Shinpiden Japanese Reiki Workshop Manual* by Richard R. Rivard and Tom Rigler.

Work hard and be kind to others.

Gassho and repeat them in your mind
  at the beginning and the end of each day.

Usui Reiki Ryoho—Improve your mind and body.

FOUNDER, MIKAO USUI

Consider the promise of the original Usui precepts: happiness and the miraculous healing for all diseases. Notice the invitation to recite them like morning and evening prayers, setting and renewing intention. Compare this translation of the precepts with the version that follows, commonly presented to Reiki students in the West:

Just for today, do not anger.
Just for today, do not worry.
Just for today, be grateful.
Just for today, do an honest day's work.
Just for today, be kind to all living things.

An eight-year-old student once asked me why we say, "just for today," again and again. I told her that we have no control over our behavior in the past, nor can we be certain of our actions in the future. The present moment presents us with the opportunity to choose how we respond to the events in our lives, as they unfold.

We may choose to remain calm, rather than respond with violence or temper. We can choose to trust, rather than becoming lost in anguished thoughts about the difficulties in our lives. We can practice being thankful from dawn to day's end and not exhaust the reasons to be grateful. We can choose to do our best and to work with integrity, no matter what others around us choose, and feel the satisfaction of accomplishment. We can find opportunities everywhere to be kind, and to enjoy the reward of healthy, fulfilling relationships with others, with our world, with ourselves.

The Reiki principles, as I was taught them and as I pass them on to my

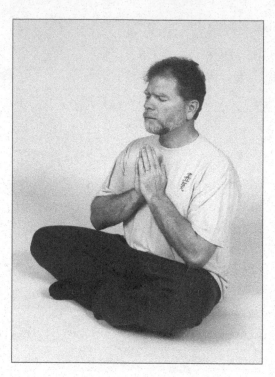

Gassho is a natural beginning and ending for meditation on the Reiki principles.

students, are reminders of our power to choose to respond to the events of our lives in ways that support health, well-being, and happiness. Since ours is not a culture that teaches us much about managing our emotions, the Reiki principles can provoke thought and invite us to claim the fullness of our humanity.

HONORING ALL LINEAGES

Our inheritance as Reiki practitioners is extraordinary. To each of us is transmitted the ability to bring healing. As channels for universal life-force energy, the healing that we can call forth and transfer to others is virtually limitless, for we tap an infinite Source.

While differences in training and proficiency may seem of paramount importance to some, overcoming the focus on differences brings a sense of unity, peace, and healing. We may experience this in the microcosm of a one-to-one relationship with a practitioner whose training is unlike our own, or on a much greater scale, as we join with practitioners of different levels and many different lineages to engage in global healing. In honoring all lineages we give ourselves the opportunity to practice tolerance, to recognize the power and the joy of shared purpose, and to participate in raising global consciousness.

Sharing knowledge across lineages offers practitioners the chance to learn more about the original history of Reiki, the many traditional techniques, and the evolution of those techniques to their present form. Learning about non-traditional techniques has value, too, as they often develop for a reason: something that has been lost over time is recognized and replaced by something new. In joining together to learn across lineages, we honor the universality of the energy—Spirit-guided, intelligent, dynamic, supportive of individual and shared spiritual growth.

PRAYER AND MEDITATION

A Reiki friend who knew I had begun to teach the Reiki and Intuition workshop presented me with a quotation from author and public speaker Wayne Dyer: "If prayer is you talking with God, intuition is God talking with you." Meditation has been defined in a related way: when we pray, we talk to God; when we meditate, we listen to God. Talking to God and listening to God are wonderful ways to prepare for a conversation with God or Spirit or Source, which is one of the many forms intuition—inner teaching—can take.

While people who are members of a church, synagogue, mosque, meeting, or temple learn at an early age to pray, those who have not been brought up in an organized religion, or who have rejected it, may feel somewhat uncertain how to pray. While it is easy to adopt a prayer, such as the Lord's Prayer, or the Prayer of Jabez, or the Unity Prayer, when we begin talking to God, it is often more comforting to use our own words. Yet how do we begin and what should we say?

Most of us, in the silence of our minds, talk to ourselves all day: "Oh, I forgot to pick up my dry cleaning at lunchtime! I'll have to get it on the way home from work . . . Why is Bob spending so much time hanging out in Sylvia's cubicle? . . . Here's a message that the day care center called. 'Alison coming down with a cold. Please pick her up early.' How can I? . . . What a sunset! Look how those last rays are shining through the red leaves on that maple tree . . .", and so on and so on. One way to pray is simply to stop talking to ourselves for a moment or two and talk instead to a higher power: "God, I need to pick Alison up early from the day care center. Please help me find a way to take care of my little girl. Thank you."

Does God or Spirit—that higher power—listen? The best way to discover the answer to this question is to say a prayer and see what happens. Sometimes the outcome we hope for is not the one that is for the highest good. If that is the case, our prayer won't be answered in the way we would like. Is that a reason to stop praying? No. The spiritual discipline of prayer has many rewards, not least of which is that prayer brings healing, a benefit any Reiki practitioner can appreciate.

Meditation also offers healing benefits, as studies made by practitioners of Transcendental Meditation have ascertained. The calming, quieting effects of focusing within, becoming still, are transforming. Although there are many books on meditation and many teachers of meditation, this practice, too, is simple and can be learned on your own. It requires deliberately stopping the motion of the day, removing attention from the emotions of the day, and becoming aware of the pulse and rhythm of life within us. Practitioners of Transcendental Meditation use a mantra, a word composed of sacred sounds, and silently chant it to still the mind. However, any word that appeals to you can be used: kindness, love, joy, the name of a Reiki symbol. Another way to meditate, shared by Zen Buddhist priest and Reiki Master Hyakuten Inamoto at the Usui Reiki Ryoho International Conference in 2002, is to quiet yourself, slow your breathing, and count each breath (each inhalation and exhalation) in a cycle that builds progressively from 1 to 5 or 10, and then begin again (1, 1-2, 1-2-3, 1-2-3-4, 1-2-3-4-5, then back to 1). Whenever you lose count, start the cycle again. This cultivates inner stillness, focused attention, and peace of mind.

Creative visualization and guided visualizations offer another way to enter the inner world. Yoga practitioners may learn to meditate on the chakras, consciously opening, closing, and balancing them; or they may be taught how to safely raise the kundalini energy that travels along the column of the spine. Tai chi, qi gong, and aikido offer moving meditations. Walking a labyrinth invites contemplation, as does focusing on a mandala.

Reiki also offers a way to enter a meditative state with ease. As soon as practitioners place their hands in position and universal life-force energy starts to flow into them and through them, tension leaves and calm comes in. The energy itself feels so good as it enters at the crown of the head and flows into the core of the body, radiating outward, that it naturally catches our attention, centering us and grounding us. If we choose to close our eyes and to see with the inner eye, we may be dazzled by a field of purple light, sparkling with golden points of energy that shimmer and soothe and heal. Could any invitation to become quiet and look within be more appealing?

Of course, we are not able to give every Reiki treatment our full attention. When we use our hands to bring healing to a coworker who has a headache, we are more likely to end up chatting about a project than quietly meditating on Reiki light. Sometimes, however, we may claim the time to do self-treatment without any distractions, and when we do client treatment, we should eliminate distractions for the client's sake. This affords us the opportunity to become quiet and fully present to the flow of Reiki energy.

THE PRACTICE OF CREATIVITY

Carl Jung, the most famous student of Sigmund Freud, wrote many books describing his theories of the development of the mind and consciousness. He observed that artists of all kinds seem to have easier access to the subconscious than people in less creative professions. Allowing ourselves to be creative lets us practice the skill of accessing our own subconscious mind and higher self. This can make the task of connecting the subconscious mind and higher self of the client, as we do intuitive Reiki, a much easier one.

Creativity, like intuition and the ability to heal through touch, is natural to all human beings. It offers us another way to go within, to connect to the self and to Spirit, to explore the sacred journey of our lives. When we allow ourselves to be creative, we discover what we value and what all human beings have valued through all time: childhood, the passage into manhood or womanhood, love and marriage, giving birth, suffering loss, gaining wisdom, experiencing death. Such universal experiences are symbolized across cultures in archetypal forms, accessible to us all through what Jung called the collective unconscious. When we surprise ourselves with our own creative vision, it is sometimes because we have expressed more than our personal feelings at this moment of time; we have explored and tapped the depths of our humanity and created something that is not only personally meaningful, but meaningful to all.

Yet most creative expression begins with a simple intention to express our feelings, clarify our thoughts, deepen our understanding of the issues that are of concern to us in our own lives. Sketching, painting, sculpting, sewing, composing, playing music, dancing, doing crafts, journaling, and all other forms of creative expression offer us the chance to raise to conscious awareness our sadness, our confusion, our joy. Claiming our creativity is a gentle way to open a door to the secrets that we, too often, keep from ourselves: heart's desire, soul's purpose, forgotten memories. Whatever we create, like dream imagery or intuitive impressions, can help us to become more aware of our need for healing. By outwardly representing our inner feelings we may view them with more objectivity and begin the healing process.

Although there are many good books about creativity, Julia Cameron's *The Artist's Way* deserves special mention as an important and helpful resource. Soon after the book was first published, Artist's Way workshops were started all over the country by individuals who wanted to use the techniques she recommends to grow creatively and who wanted to claim the support of a community. There are still Artist's Way workshops that are ongoing and open to newcomers. You may want to see if there is one in your area, or you may want to start one yourself.

JOURNALING

The blank page of a journal is like a backyard covered with fresh snow. It's up to you whether you will simply enjoy the view out the window or go out and play:

make a snowman, make a snow angel, go sledding. A journal doesn't even have to be in spiral-bound notebook form, although many people find this convenient. Looseleaf pages, colored paper, newsprint, and a blank computer screen all present the same sense of possibility.

Sometimes people think of a journal as a diary and wonder what they might have to say of interest, even to themselves, day after day. Liberating yourself from that concept will go a long way toward freeing you to express your creativity, heal, grow, and become who you are meant to be. There is no wrong way to keep a journal, and reveling in the freedom to misspell, to ignore grammar, to write in the margins, can be fun. In fact, writing each word that comes into your head without attempting to control or order your thoughts, recording the "stream of consciousness," can bring personal revelations and deeper self-understanding.

A journal can be home to poems, stories, snatches of conversation overheard on a bus, sketches, "to do" lists, grocery lists, affirmations, daydreams, goals. It can also be used to record dreams and fragments of dreams each morning, prayers and intentions, conversations with God, and letters to angels. For inspiration you might read Natalie Goldberg's *Writing Down the Bones*; Patricia Garfield's *Creative Dreaming*; Donald Neale Walsch's *Conversations with God;* and Barbara Mark's and Trudy Griswold's *Angelspeake* and *The Angelspeake Book of Prayer and Healing*.

DIVINING

While learning how to read tarot cards or runes can offer exercise in understanding images and symbols and interpreting them accurately, these activities are best practiced with the conscious intention to connect to Spirit and ask for truthful, helpful, loving guidance. Many people try these methods at some point during their lives, either through self-study, class instruction, or receiving a reading. They may go to a tarot card reader or a psychic at a holistic fair, pay the fee, and see what happens. Will the reading be on target? Or will some of the information be right on the nose and the rest be so unbelievable that the whole experience is dismissed as nonsense and a waste of money?

The Bible warns against false prophets. Are tarot card readers and psychics just that? While there are charlatans and gimmicky fortune tellers, most intuitive readers are professional, ethical, and feel a spiritual calling to offer guidance and healing. The best intuitive readers acknowledge that the most reliable source for guidance is within each individual. They do not "guarantee results," because they recognize the power of individual free will and know that any future events they glimpse are possibilities, perhaps probabilities, but not predetermined. They also present whatever intuitive impressions they receive in a way that is uplifting, encouraging, and empowering to the client.

This is one of the ways to recognize true guidance, whether it is offered to us through a reader, comes to us in meditation or after prayer, or flows into conscious awareness as we do Reiki on a client or ourselves: it is inspiring and healing.

Years ago a dear friend who worked as a professional intuitive reader taught me a simple way to ask for guidance that I still use today. Go to your bookshelf; close your eyes and quiet your mind. Ask Spirit to guide you, focus on a question or concern, and then reach for a book. Hold it in your hands for a moment with the awareness that Spirit, who is all-knowing, knows the contents of the book. Then open it and see where your eye falls on the page. Read and discover the power of Spirit to speak to you through any medium.

Will this method work if you don't take it seriously? Probably not. Just like a friend who doesn't like being dismissed or ignored, Spirit isn't likely to offer you guidance if you are not sincere in your desire to receive it. Will this method work if you are choosing from a bookshelf full of medical or engineering textbooks or software instruction guides? Again, perhaps not. Spiritual books and scripture, metaphysical books, and self-help books are written to offer guidance, so you may most easily find the answer you seek in their pages.

ONE AFTERNOON

The spring after my mother died I gave myself a lot of solitary time to grieve and to think. For the previous three years all my dreams had been put on hold so that I could be with her, talk to her, care for her. I felt blessed to have been at her side so many days and nights and at the moment of her death. Yet I felt a need to recall myself to my own life, so I spent an afternoon journaling, purging myself of pent-up frustration as I remembered goals I had given up and wondered what was still possible. "Lots of dreams," I wrote. "I've always had lots of dreams. Yet I've managed to manifest so few," I complained on paper. I continued to write until I felt emptied of negativity. Then, following another impulse, I drove to the Barnes & Noble bookstore in nearby Allentown. Here I could drink a cappuccino and page through a magazine, and perhaps find more inspiration to write.

As I waited in the long queue of customers I picked up a book on the display table near the counter: Robin S. Sharma's *The Monk Who Sold His Ferrari*. I opened the book at random (so I thought) and read:

> I'm not saying you have to leave the legal profession tomorrow. You will, however, have to start taking risks. Shake up your life a bit. Get rid of the cobwebs. Take the road less traveled. Most people live within the confines of their comfort zone. Yogi Raman was the first person to explain to me that the best thing you can do for yourself is regularly move beyond it. This is the way to lasting personal mastery and to realize the true potential of your human endowments.

Hmmm . . . , I thought. This couldn't possibly be meant for me, could it? I read on to discover on the facing page the monk's recommendation to practice a four-thousand-year-old meditation called The Heart of the Rose. My heart quickened a bit, my interest captured. This could not possibly be the same meditation that had come to me, as I did Reiki on myself, a few months ago. Or could it?

In fact, it was, with one essential difference. In the meditation that I had "discovered" intuitively, a focus on an imaginary rose was sufficient to bring a sense of calm, a renewed awareness of beauty, an appreciation of life. The Tibetan meditation described in Robin Sharma's book was more grounded: the practitioner was to contemplate a real rose with presence of mind and appreciation. The promised result was a quality of calm, a greater sense of control over the mind, and the awakening of joy.

Why did I find myself with this book in hand, reminding me gently and easily of a meditation practice I had become aware of through intuitive Reiki, loved for its simplicity, practiced briefly, and let go? How was it that I found myself in this bookstore, beside the "Humorous, Helpful, and Odd" display of books, picking up *The Monk Who Sold His Ferrari* out of the thirty or so books spread out on the table? How was it that I opened the book to exactly those pages that reminded me that I would need to be willing to leave my "comfort zone" to effect real change in my life—and suggested a familiar meditation?

Did I need a reminder to do meditation? "Yes," said the quiet inner voice in my head. Did I need encouragement to take risks? "Yes, again," the voice said. Was this whole event in my life divinely guided and orchestrated? "Yes." And then came this instruction, which I recorded in my journal: "You need to let people know that when you open up to guidance, it comes both from 'within' and 'without'—for All-That-Is is expressing what is guidance for each one."

SUGGESTIONS FOR PRACTITIONERS

Claim the gifts of the present in your own life. While workshops and books can provide inspiration and instruction, you have available within you all the resources you need to become more intuitive and to grow spiritually—as long as you are willing to ask Spirit for a little help.

Practice Reiki with an appreciation of the strong connection to Spirit that it creates. As you feel universal life-force energy flowing through you, notice how it centers you, inviting you to attend to your inner life. Be open to receiving guidance in whatever form it comes to you, and be humble and patient enough to wait if guidance does not come immediately. Be willing to accept that there are times that we are not meant to know the answers, when we are meant to learn to trust.

Continue to practice Reiki. Be willing to deepen your commitment to service. Learn to pray or to meditate. Use whatever spiritual and metaphysical knowledge you have acquired along the way. Open your heart to receive and be willing to accept whatever blessings are offered to you in the present moment.

NOW YOU

Dance, sing, write, draw. Use whatever form of creative expression appeals to you to express the feelings that you hold inside—and let them go, knowing that you open the way for deeper feelings to emerge. In discovering that you can choreograph a dance, compose music, pen a poem, sketch a landscape, bake an amazing apple pie, you will become more aware of your power to envision and to co-create, with Spirit's help, your own life.

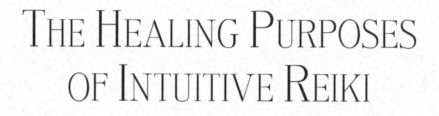

THE HEALING PURPOSES
OF INTUITIVE REIKI

Intuition serves to direct us to our highest good in countless ways: it can suggest to us the least trafficked road home, reducing our chances of being in an accident or being stressed out by delays; it can prompt us to visit a particular place at a particular time, so that we encounter an old friend in need of an attentive listener; it can urge us to question something that others take for granted—the safety of a particular swimming hole, for example—revealing a hidden danger to all; it can guide us to move to a new location or a new job, where we soon meet a life partner. More simply stated, intuition can help ease our journey, enhance our sense of well-being, guide us to life's pleasures, protect us from life's dangers, find right work, help us balance work and play, perform with perfect timing, serve our communities in meaningful ways, and connect to soul friends and soulmates. When we listen to intuition we listen to the voice of the soul, which steadily, gently guides us toward greater health and well-being, fulfillment and happiness.

When intuition, which serves to direct us to our highest good, is accessed and used during Reiki healing, which is offered for the highest good, the healing that occurs can be profound, because it is so strongly and intentionally aligned with the wisdom of the soul. When a client has a chronic physical complaint or a progressive, debilitating illness, there are often old emotional issues that must be addressed before deep, complete, permanent healing can occur. Intuition used during Reiki treatment of such a client can help the client to identify emotions that have been repressed and that need to be released; negative thoughts that have become habitual and that need to be replaced; people, places, or situations that have become draining or damaging and that have been denied—and that now need to be acknowledged and forgiven before forward progress can be made.

When a client receives an injury in an accident or contracts an acute infection, there is often an analogous emotional event that has served as a catalyst, making the client feel more anxious and, therefore, more accident-prone, or depressing the client and lowering the immune system response. Again, intuitive impressions that arise while treating such clients with Reiki can suggest the original cause of the injury or infection. If the client can simply be encouraged to reflect on this cause and process the feelings that it evoked, the physical healing that occurs during the treatment will be accompanied by conscious emotional healing, which is empowering to the client, enabling the client to integrate the healing that has occurred on all levels so that it is both more effective and more enduring.

When a client is basically well and receiving Reiki for relaxation, intuitive Reiki can offer encouragement, reassurance, reinforcement for positive lifestyle choices already made, validation, clarification, guidance. Intuitive impressions may arise that relieve the client's stress and tension by inviting discussion. This airing of concerns can help the client to feel more at ease, soothing the heart and calming the mind. A healthy client may also have old wounds—physical, mental, emotional, spiritual—that are incompletely healed; these wounds may originate as far back as early childhood or farther back, in another lifetime. Intuitive impressions that arise during a Reiki treatment may help the client to identify such old injuries and old issues still in need of healing.

Of course, because every human being is enormously complex, a client can be well enough to lead a normal life and yet be compromised by illness or injury at the same time. As a result, the intuitive impressions that arise during a Reiki session may serve several purposes, some of them revealing what is in need of further healing, some of them reinforcing healthy choices already made, some guiding the client toward a happier, healthier future. For any client, well or ill, there is always the possibility of intuitive impressions arising that are indicative of some future issue or opportunity (since to Spirit—and to the Reiki energy, which comes from Spirit—all time is now).

The result is that, for a practitioner who uses intuitive Reiki, a kaleidoscopic array of images and impressions may arise during the treatment of a client, or a few key images and impressions may arise, or none at all. (Note: Just as what you perceive while listening to your hands depends on the client's need for healing, what you perceive as a practitioner while "listening to your intuition" depends on the client's need for healing—especially emotional and mental healing—and the client's willingness to communicate this need.) The intuitive impressions that arise during a Reiki treatment may seem to serve a wide variety of purposes, yet all serve the fundamental spiritual purpose of directing the client to his or her highest good and supporting the practitioner's intention to offer Reiki for the highest good.

HEALING AN OLD INJURY

As Reiki Master Kay Sivel fulfilled the final requirement for her training by assisting for the third time at a Reiki II class, she shared this story: "Recently I was invited over to a friend's house for a get-together. There were four of us, and we all got on really well. I offered to do Reiki on my friend, who said she would be glad to have a treatment. So I went out to my car and brought in my table and set it up. I treated her and then I treated one of the other women.

"The whole time, the conversation never stopped. We just kept talking and laughing. After I completed the hand positions on the woman's lower chest and abdomen, I found myself with my hands on this woman's knees. Then, when I felt a shift in the flow of the Reiki energy, I moved my hands—again, without thinking—to cover her left shin. This is not a position that I normally use, but my hands just went there naturally, and they became quite warm.

"After a few minutes the woman broke into the conversation to tell me that the Reiki felt so good—and that I was right over the place where she had broken her leg. I had no idea that she had broken her leg. I had never met her before in my life—yet the Reiki energy guided my hands there.

"I found this experience really amazing. It showed me what can happen when I just relax, let the Reiki flow, and listen to my hands. The guidance just comes naturally."

CONFIRMING A NEED FOR MEDICAL TREATMENT

Shortly after my first book, *Traditional Reiki for Our Times,* was published, I gave a presentation on Reiki at the local branch of the Bucks County Free Library. Ever since I worked there the summer between my junior and senior year of high school I have felt close to the librarians. They were very pleased to host an event to support me as a local author. They were also curious about Reiki, so they slipped in and out of the presentation, which was held in a conference room that opened off the main room of the library.

As I described Reiki to the audience of about thirty people, I invited individuals to come up to the front of the room, sit in a chair, and receive Reiki on their head, neck, shoulders—wherever the sensations in my hands intensified, indicating a need for healing. As I continued to talk about Reiki and to tell stories of my experience, several people took advantage of my invitation and then described what they felt to the audience. Toward the end of my presentation I noticed a gentleman in the back of the room, writing notes frantically on a yellow legal pad. As I finished doing Reiki on the shoulders of the woman in the chair, I asked him, "Are you a reporter?"

"Yes," he admitted. He was a reporter for *The Morning Call.*

"Well, then, you should come on up and experience Reiki!" I said, smiling, welcoming him with a wave of my hand.

He set down his legal pad, walked to the front of the room, and took a seat, looking a bit uncertain. I scanned his energy field and noticed a sudden focal point of intensification on the left side of his face, over his back upper teeth.

"Is something going on with your teeth?" I asked. "Have you been having some dental work perhaps? Or do you need some dental work?"

He jumped and looked up at me with suspicion. "How do you know that?"

I explained that I could feel a change in sensation in my hands as I moved them through his energy field in that area.

He said that he had been having some trouble with a back tooth on that side and his dentist had advised him to have a root canal, but the work hadn't been done yet. "And you say that anyone can learn to do this?" he asked.

"Yes, anyone can learn to do Reiki and become sensitive to the changes in their hands." He didn't seem convinced, but he did notice that the pain in that area begin to diminish. He ended up writing two positive articles about Reiki, recommending that readers check it out.

MONITORING A HEALTH ISSUE

Ann Pedersen, who learned Reiki in spring 2005, did so with the thought that it might help her better care for her two athletic children. During this small class I had the opportunity to be her client for the supervised practice session, and then to give her a Reiki treatment in return. Ann seemed to be in very good health, so the energy in my hands in Basic I positions 1, 2, 3 (over the lower chest and abdomen) was unremarkable—what I have experienced in treating someone who is well, but coping with everyday stress. In Basic I position 4, at the V of the pelvic cradle, the warmth and tingling I was experiencing in my hands became considerably more intense. I tilted my head, as if "listening" harder. Ann noticed my concentration.

"What is it?" she asked. "What is it that you sense?"

"Well, I don't think that there's anything to be alarmed about," I said, wanting to reassure her. "There's just a lot of energy flowing into this area—and it feels different than the sensations that might indicate hormonal changes from your monthly cycle. It's hard to describe. It almost feels as though the tissue under my hands is thickened in some way—I guess it could be just as a result of childbirth." She looked at me with some concern. "I really don't think that it's anything to worry about, but the way to make sure is to go to your doctor and get it checked out. Then you'll have peace of mind about it."

She nodded. "I'll do that."

I continued the treatment on her head and back, completing it with Reiki on the soles of her feet, to help distribute the healing energy throughout her body and to help her feel balanced and grounded. We continued with the class, and at the end of the day I certified Ann as Reiki I and congratulated her on her accomplishment. "Please stay in touch," I told her. "Let me know if you have any questions or if you just want to share an experience of Reiki."

Several weeks passed before I heard from her again. She wrote to thank me and enclosed a copy of the results of an MRI test her gynecologist had prescribed. The results of the test showed a small myoma, a thickening of the middle of the uterus on one side—nothing to be alarmed about, but something her gynecologist will continue to monitor over time.

What was curious about this experience for me was that she thanked me for listening to my intuition, describing my impression and recommending that she see a doctor. To my way of thinking, I had simply listened to my hands and described what I could sense through my hands. The experience helped me understand that intuitive impressions can occur, as healing occurs, in the flow of the Reiki energy. Whether we sense such impressions with our hands or with another part of our energy anatomy, we are sensing something that is given to us for the purpose of healing on all levels.

CLARIFYING CONCERNS, LETTING GO OF WORRY

My client, a tall, willowy woman in excellent health from her many years as a yoga practitioner and teacher, lay on her back in a tee shirt and sweatpants, her eyes closed, her breathing relaxed. She had asked me to give her a Reiki treatment using her own bodywork table, which she keeps set up in the sunroom of her house on the Delaware River. Now, in late June, the sunroom was partially shaded by the branches of trees leafing out, the tall, screened windows were open to catch the breeze, and a fan turned in quiet, lazy circles overhead.

As I treated her on the front of her torso, the Reiki energy flowed with steady warmth but without dramatic intensity over any area. This made sense in terms of what I knew of my client. Not only is this baby boomer a yoga teacher, but she is also a retired physical therapist and a Reiki Master herself. She is wise enough to take good care of herself: she eats a healthy diet, gets more than adequate exercise, takes appropriate nutritional supplements, and she treats herself daily with Reiki. Once a month, to help her cope with stress during a difficult time in her life, she calls another Reiki practitioner to do a full treatment.

Like many people, this woman carries stress in her neck, shoulders, and lower back. During this particular treatment she also presented the fading red mark of a recent deer tick bite just above her collarbone, and she was still taking a prescribed course of antibiotics for Lyme disease. When I moved around the table to treat my client's head, I was not surprised to find that the Reiki energy flowed with greater intensity there.

As I am trained to do when working at the head, I drew the first and second symbols in the sequence recommended by my teacher and proceeded, in the silence of my mind, to "chat" with my client.

"How are you feeling this afternoon?"

"Oh, I'm just fine, thank you. I'm really enjoying the Reiki." (Just as many people respond to an inquiry after their health with a brief, polite reply that gives no details, so, too, many Reiki clients initially respond to a practitioner's silent question in the same way. More details usually follow, if the practitioner is patient, just as they did during this afternoon session.)

Silently, I asked another question: "Are there any areas of your physical body that need some extra attention and healing today?"

Suddenly, behind my closed eyes, I saw my client just as if I were looking at her with my eyes open: she lay relaxed on her back, her legs stretched out, on the bodywork table. Now, however, my attention was strongly drawn to the inside of her left knee and down her left calf, then to the arches of her feet.

Mentally, I said, "Thank you for showing me those areas. I promise I will give them some Reiki later on during the treatment." Then I prompted her with another question. "Are there any other issues or concerns that are affecting the way you are feeling today?"

With my mind's eye I saw my client stepping lightly but carefully over a small stream in the woods. As she watched her footing I heard her say, "Oh, I'll cross that stream when I come to it." My intuitive feeling was that this image was related to a work opportunity she had described to me earlier as we caught up on her news. I broke the silence in the sunroom to describe the image to my client, who was relaxed but awake, and asked if she understood it.

"Yes, I do," she said. "The opportunity that I have been offered to teach at this other yoga center is one that will be open to me for some time. I don't have to decide today, although I wish I felt less conflicted about what to do." The problem, she explained, was this: "I love the students that I have now and I feel very loyal to them. I don't want to leave them, but this is an attractive opportunity—and I have been asking Spirit to give me some new career opportunities, some new possibilities. I would really like to be able to teach Reiki, as well as yoga, and I might be able to do both at this new yoga center."

To comfort my client I explained that many of my own Reiki students had remained within my circle and gradually become my dearest friends—my spiritual family—over the years. I didn't see any reason why she should worry that her present yoga students might feel abandoned or want to abandon her. She could invite them to stay connected to her through friendship.

Yes, she said, she could do that.

"Is there any reason that you couldn't continue teaching your current yoga students and also take this position?"

"No," she said. "In fact, I plan to continue with my present teaching schedule and gradually take on more classes at this new yoga center. I think that eventually I would have to settle on teaching in one location, simply because the center where I now teach and the new center are in opposite directions, miles apart."

"And do you feel as though you have some time to think over this decision?" I asked, remembering the intuitive impression I had received.

"Yes, I have a little bit of time. I don't have to decide today." She sighed and settled herself again, relaxing more deeply into the flow of Reiki.

I closed my eyes and resumed our inner dialogue: "Are there any other issues of concern to you today?" Suddenly I saw her as a young child looking up at herself as an older woman, who restrained a little pug-nosed, long-eared dog on a leash. The child looked on with concern as the woman yelled at the little dog, trying to get it to heel. However, instead of saying, "Heel," she was saying, "Toe the line!" She seemed very angry and harsh, and completely focused on the dog. She seemed not to notice the child, who now shrank back in horror at this show of temper.

Softly, I said my client's name and asked if I might share another impression with her. When she agreed, I cautioned her that the impression was complicated and it would take me a little time to describe it in full. When I finished I asked whether she understood it. She said that she wasn't sure, so I told her about the feelings I associated with each part of the image. "Because I am seeing you at once as both a child and as an older woman, I am wondering whether the image is connected to your childhood, and perhaps to your feelings as a child about your mother and her behaviors. What was she like?"

My client explained to me that both of her parents were harsh disciplinarians, and her mother, unlike most women of the 1950s, had a full-time career. When anything or anyone interfered with her work, she would lash out. (This was the first clue that we weren't done discussing my client's new career opportunity.)

"Did she try to be a full-time homemaker as well?"

"Yes, she did."

"Did she get angry in response to feeling overwhelmed or tired?"

"Yes, that was her pattern," my client agreed.

"Do you ever get angry when you are overwhelmed or overtired?"

"Yes, absolutely."

"Is it possible that you are concerned about taking on too much by accepting this position at the new yoga center, feeling overwhelmed, and then lashing out at people you care for?"

"Yes, it is quite possible. It is one of the reasons that I feel some pressure to decide between the two positions, rather than trying to do both."

"Let's see if we can make any sense of the dog." I reviewed the details of the image with my client. The older version of herself had been yelling at the dog to "toe the line." I realized, with a chuckle, that she had mentioned that the new center was in Line Lexington. Could this message be a pun on the name of the town?

It could, my client decided. "One of my concerns," she said, "is that there are several people who will be involved in running this center. I want to be able to line up everyone's support for what I want to do and then I just want to do it."

"Are you concerned that you might have to be more forceful or assertive than might feel comfortable to you in order to gain that support?"

"It's an issue that's been in the back of my mind," she said. "Now that I am more aware of it, I can think it through carefully and then make my decision. I have some time. . . ." She smiled, still with her eyes closed, as if asleep, and relaxed even more into the flow of Reiki as she consciously let go of this concern.

When I invited her to resume our inner dialogue, she was silent, content with what had been accomplished in terms of her emotional and mental healing. I continued to treat her with Reiki until I had completed the treatment of all the formal positions, and then I placed my hands on the inside of her left knee and calf, as she had requested. I finished the treatment by grounding her with Reiki energy to the soles of her feet.

ROAD SIGN: THIS WAY TO HAPPINESS

Natalie James, a Reiki Master and massage therapist who works at a holistic center in Ambler, Pennsylvania, shared this story with me about an impression that came to her as she treated a regular client who had returned recently from a trip.

"Last year, when doing intuitive Reiki on one of my clients, I saw a Ho-Ho, one of those chocolate cake and cream snacks so many of us found in our lunch boxes as kids. Although I felt a little embarrassed to admit what had popped into my mind (maybe my client would think I was just hungry!), I blurted it out to her anyway. At the end of the session, when I asked her if any of the images I had described during the treatment meant anything to her, she honed in on the Ho-Ho.

"She said she thought of Ho-Hos as something sweet, with black embracing white. It turned out that she had just come back from the most heartwarming, sweet experience of her life—in Africa, where she was welcomed, respected, loved, and embraced by the black community. She had done missionary work there, helping out at an orphanage. The whole experience had been so positive for her that she had already decided that she would go back in 2005. As a footnote, she came back from this year's trip wearing an engagement ring, given to her by a man she met last year. They are very much in love and look forward to a life together. So she was embraced by more than just the community!"

IT'S OKAY TO HAVE FUN

Although I am living my dream of teaching Reiki, I juggle responsibilities seven days a week. Occasionally I find myself thinking about how other people live and I pine to have some good, old-fashioned fun: a hayride on an autumn night, a ski trip with dinner in front of a fireplace in the lodge, a Sunday afternoon in an art museum. To that end I sometimes study continuing education catalogs and think about how to fit a jewelry-making or Italian language class into my schedule. Last spring one class that caught my interest was goat milk soap-making. I am as fond of fine, fresh-scented soap as anyone, and I found the idea of using soap I had made for a leisurely bath appealing; but what really captured my attention in this particular class advertisement was that the soap-making process would begin with milking a goat! The class would meet for two evening sessions, and the price was quite reasonable. Should I sign up?

As I drove to a Reikishare in a nearby town I mulled over the possibility. Could I spare two evenings from my schedule for the class? Would it be fun to milk a goat or frightening? How would my soap turn out? Once I arrived at the Reikishare I put all this out of my mind and occupied myself with setting up chairs and bodywork tables, greeting people and catching up on their news.

An hour and a half or so later, when I lay on the table, eyes closed, relaxed, enjoying the Reiki energy I was receiving from those gathered around, Reiki Master Lynn Thiel, who had her hands over my ears, burst out laughing. "I don't believe this!" she said. "I see a goat! Do you have any idea what this means?"

I patted her hand. "It's okay, Lynn. Your intuition is right on." I explained to her that just that morning I had been looking at a continuing education catalog and debating whether or not I should take a course in goat milk soap-making.

She laughed. "Well, I think you should take the class. I think you would find it a lot of fun."

Fun, I thought. Ah. . . . "Okay, I'll call the school this week to see about signing up," I promised.

I did just that, and learned to my regret that the goat milk soap-making class was already filled with the maximum number of students the teacher would accept. Reiki had offered me guidance, and I had attempted to honor the guidance by acting on it—but not quickly enough. This opportunity is one that I look forward to claiming another time.

COMMUNICATING SUPPORT IN THE PRESENT

Early in my distant-healing practice a close friend asked me to send Reiki to his grandmother, who was feeling low because she had fallen on a patch of ice and broken an ankle. Now she was confined indoors, through the cold gray days of February, while her husband, a retired country doctor, hovered over her. In addition, a specialist had just diagnosed her with Parkinson's disease, although she vehemently rejected this doctor's opinion. She was so weak and so upset by this bleak turn of events that my friend wanted to find some way to cheer her up. Could I send her Reiki healing and see if I received any guidance he might use?

Eager to help him, I sat down, calmed myself, and began to send her distant healing. I was able to comfort him by sharing my impression that there was still some time—at least a couple of years—in which to visit with her, share stories, make new memories. For the moment she would be cheered by a visit from him and a bunch of daffodils. If she could be prevailed upon to let him cook, then he should make a dinner that included fresh steamed asparagus with melted butter, and for dessert, fresh ripe strawberries. All these gestures would tell her, as words might not, that spring was on its way and, with it, a sense of renewed physical energy and hope.

He called her moments after I described these impressions and asked if he might come to see her. She invited him out that afternoon. The bouquet of bright yellow daffodils that he gave her surprised and cheered her. The dinner he cooked for her, light and nurturing, encouraged her to eat with more enthusiasm than she had in many days. She took from it not only physical sustenance but heart's comfort. As winter slowly yielded to spring's gentle warmth, she grew stronger and carried herself forward, supported by a cane, with dignity and no trembling in her fingers.

ENCOURAGEMENT FOR THE FUTURE

At a Reiki Masters' share in the fall of 2003, my students and I joined together to send distant healing to planet Earth, and to individuals and situations of concern to each of those present. Finally, we sent Reiki to one another, with each practitioner treating the person seated to the right. Then we shared our impressions. Colleen Lavdar, a personable museum director and a recently certified Reiki Master, was astounded that I offered her the words "electronic newspaper," which had floated into my mind with a few other impressions as I sat, eyes closed, sending her Reiki.

"I can't believe you said that! I was talking just this morning to my husband about how much I would like to put together an electronic newsletter for my Reiki students. I've only just thought of the idea."

I smiled at her. "Well, perhaps it is a good one, and you should make it a goal and pursue it to completion."

"It's likely to be a while before I put the first issue together, but I'll certainly keep it under consideration."

The stream of subtle energy that is the flow of Reiki had shone its light on a future possibility. The client connected with the idea, current in her thought, not yet manifested in reality, and recognized her free will to follow through or not.

SUGGESTIONS FOR PRACTITIONERS

Consider the possibility that the world exists in a state of consciousness, as pervasive and sustaining as the air that we breathe. Within it are our perceptions of reality, our daydreams, fantasies, hopes, expectations, desires, beliefs, prayers, positive and negative thoughts, fears, frustrations, anxieties, nightmares. Within it is all that we think of as the past, the present, the future. Within it also is the awareness of one another both as other and as the same.

When we ask for intuitive guidance while doing Reiki, we ask for those perceptions, those thoughts, those feelings that are for the client's highest good to rise on the energy, to surface in our individual consciousness in a form that will allow us to offer them to the client for consideration and contemplation, sometimes during the treatment, but more often at a later time. When we ask for intuitive guidance while doing Reiki on ourselves, we ask for the same healing gifts from Spirit.

Consider this possibility, and become more peaceful with the healing purposes intuitive Reiki serves. Then review your own experiences as a Reiki practitioner. Has information that you received in the form of an intuitive impression—an image, a word, a scent, a tactile sensation, a feeling, a knowing—ever supported your client's healing? Has your description of an impression ever helped to reassure, encourage, bring clarity or comfort? Has a comment you made motivated a client to follow up the treatment with a visit to a physician? Be grateful that you have been able to support your client's healing by practicing Reiki in an intuitive way.

NOW YOU

Besides going to the Reiki table with an open mind and heart, ready to receive inner guidance on behalf of your client, acknowledge your own willingness to receive inner guidance by using affirmations. Here are a few you might try:

- I allow myself to see the value of intuition in my Reiki practice and understand the healing purposes intuitive Reiki serves. I ask to receive intuitive impressions as I do Reiki.

- I am an intuitive person. I am open to being guided by my intuition, I expect to be guided by my intuition, and I am grateful for the guidance I receive.
- I ask to be guided by Spirit today and every day. I am grateful for Spirit's guidance today and every day. As I feel grateful, I notice that I am being guided by Spirit more and more often.

As with all affirmations, your own wording will probably work best. Please remember to word your statements in a positive, uplifting way, as if your goal is already accomplished. Use the present tense. Remember the power of *"I am,"* which is one translation for the Hebrew name of God, to help you create healthy transformation in your life. Keep your statement simple so that it is easy to recall and repeat throughout the day. Remember to express gratitude.

While there are many ways to use affirmations, repeating them is the key to changing a behavior. You might want to write your affirmation on a post-it note and stick it on your bathroom mirror, on your car's dashboard, on your computer monitor, anywhere that you will see it often; recite your affirmation silently when you see it. Or you might write out your affirmation on an index card and read it a few times in the morning, at mid-day, and in the evening. (If you repeat your affirmation three times, three times a day, you will be adopting a time-honored pattern of prayer.) Or you might write out the affirmation on a piece of paper and simply send some Reiki energy into it, repeating the affirmation and the Reiki, as needed. Advanced practitioners can send Reiki to the affirmation they have chosen using the distant-healing symbols so that it becomes even more charged with Reiki healing, to support the expansion of their intuitive skills as a Reiki practitioner.

‚

Learning how to listen to our intuition—our inner guidance—can be as much fun to the inner child as playing hide-and-seek was for most of us once upon a time. At the start of the day ask Spirit to guide your travels (if you have the freedom to choose the route). Ask to be shown the traffic route that will gift you with the most beautiful scenery or that will allow you to reach your destination most quickly. Close your eyes and see what comes into your mind—images, words, feelings. Follow the guidance and be grateful for the beauty—or the ease—Spirit gives you. (Those who travel to busy downtowns or cities might vary this by asking to be shown the best parking place.)

When you get the hang of this "game," invite Spirit to guide you in other ways. If you are someone who makes several phone calls each day, ask Spirit to guide you to call at the perfect time to find your party in the office or at home. If you are searching for an item that you have misplaced, or someone else has misplaced, or you are in a hurry and shopping for the perfect gift, ask Spirit to show you where to find the item. See what comes to mind. You may be surprised—and very pleased—by the results.

This is a lighthearted—and practical—way to discover how willingly Spirit supports us all. Remember to say thank you to Spirit for all guidance you are given.

6

TRADITIONAL INTUITIVE
REIKI TECHNIQUES

After a few months of corresponding with me by e-mail, graduate student Candace Ferrandino registered to take Reiki I at the Dreamcatcher, a Native American gift shop in Skippack, Pennsylvania, that has a wonderful workshop space where I often teach. After the class Candace wrote to me again.

> Thank you so much for teaching me Reiki and the time that you spent sharing your knowledge and your experiences. I wanted to tell you that I had a very enlightened experience when I returned home. As I was getting out of my car, I noticed for the first time how beautiful the trees were outside my house. It looked as if the trees were illuminated. It was such a strange but wonderful experience. I sat there for a few minutes just relishing what I saw. I am thankful and truly believe that my senses were heightened from the Reiki class.

In my reply to Candace I thanked her for reminding me of something that is so fundamental to the experience of teaching, learning, and practicing Reiki that I sometimes take it for granted: it heightens our sensory perception, or, in the words of my own teacher for the basic course, "Reiki enhances the quality of life."

Reiki enlightens us, as well as empowering us to bring healing. That enlightenment, for most of us, is not a lightning bolt experience but is instead a gentle, gradual unfolding that allows us, over time, to discover our own true nature: we are "of the Spirit." We come to understand this by contemplating the experience of Reiki healing and our own role in it, which is to serve as a conduit, a channel, for universal or (more closely translated from Japanese) "Spirit-guided" life-force energy. To invite this contemplation, we are offered countless clues: the healing we ourselves experience as we treat a client; the feeling of peace that descends on us as we give Reiki to ourselves; and the myriad sensations in our hands and our perceptions of them, which may or may not match those of the client. Perhaps most telling is the curious sensation that physical boundaries have dissolved: our hands have become pure energy, the area of the client's body under our hands has become pure energy, and we are one. On the way to that extraordinary awareness (for it is not an awareness that I, at least, experience every day) are many other moments of altered perception, including the heightened sensory awareness that Candace discovered immediately following her Reiki I class.

Reiki fascinates and intrigues; it comforts and soothes; it heals in ways that are beyond our comprehension. Reiki entices us forward toward enlightenment as we are learning it, as we practice it each day, as we teach it and share our experiences with others. Because our perception is clarified and our sensory awareness heightened, we can appreciate our world made new, feel deeper gratitude, open to greater joy—and perhaps someday, in some way, acknowledge the presence of Spirit, as pervasive as energy, in all creation.

Becoming more intuitive is a natural part of this evolution. While only a handful of traditional Western lineages teach specific Reiki techniques that incorporate the use of intuition, many traditional and nontraditional Reiki Masters let their students know that yes, they can expect to become more intuitive, just as, with practice, they can expect to become more aware of the sensations of energy in their hands.

If this comment is all that you were offered in your own Reiki I class regarding intuition, do not be discouraged. As you continue to work with Reiki, the energy itself will help you to evolve to the point where you are comfortable receiving intuitive impressions as you do Reiki and you are open to receiving inner guidance in your own life. This book is intended to help you release old fears, set aside self-doubts, and claim your natural ability, enhanced by Reiki. It is Reiki practice, however, that will teach you, more effectively than any written set of instructions, how to be in the flow of the energy itself, open and receptive to any intuitive impressions that may arise.

INTUITIVE REIKI IN BASIC PRACTICE: HANDS-ON

"When you are working on a client at the bodywork table, even though you are newly attuned to Reiki and just starting to practice, you may find that your intuition brings something to mind that may be helpful or healing for the client." The small circle of Reiki I students listens attentively, their heads angled, their eyes alert.

"Reiki transforms you into a channel of healing and expands your perception of subtle energy, so that you can notice changes in the sensations in your hands and be guided by them to give the client a thorough treatment. That expansion in your perception also makes it more likely that you will receive intuitive impressions that may be of value to the client. This won't happen every time you treat a client, but it will happen occasionally—and you need to be prepared for when it does."

"How will I know when I receive an impression?" a young woman asks.

"Well, it might take a while—a bit of practice time at the bodywork table—to learn to sort out the daydreams and the stray thoughts from the true intuitive impressions, but eventually you'll be able to do it. Sometimes, though, it's easy. You will be completely focused on the flow of the Reiki energy into your hands, watching swirls of light behind your closed eyes, and all of sudden something will pop into your mind: an image of a baseball player sliding into a base, a line of melody from an old song. You'll think, 'Now where did that come from?' When you describe the impression to your client, the client will be able to identify it.

"But please remember that you can give a Reiki treatment that is truly healing to the client on many levels without receiving any intuitive impressions at all. There is nothing wrong with the treatment—or with you—if no impressions occur."

In the brief silence that follows this statement, I look at each face to make sure everyone has taken this in. Then I continue: "Intuition is a natural ability, just as sight, smell, hearing, taste, and touch are natural abilities. Intuition helps us to make sense of our inner world, just as our external senses help us make sense of the external world. Both help us find our way in life.

"Just by hearing the word *intuition* you can guess at how it functions: it offers us inner teaching. How do we learn its lessons? We pay attention to our inner life. Just as we have a set of physical senses with which to perceive the external world, so we also have a set of spiritual senses with which to perceive our inner life." I look around the circle at the students' faces, seeing curiosity and intense concentration.

"How many of you remember your dreams?" I ask. Most of the students nod. One shrugs and says, "Only once in a while."

"Have you ever noticed, as you drift off to sleep, the images that form here?" I ask, touching my fingertip to the center of my forehead. Several of the students nod. "Have you realized that when you daydream, the same thing happens?" Now they are all in agreement.

"Have you ever imagined hearing voices or music or the sound of a ball cracking against a bat or a door slamming or a teakettle boiling as you dreamed—or daydreamed?" Now some of the students are smiling. They can guess what I will say next. "If so, you have heard with your inner ears.

"We have an equivalent set of senses with which we can perceive our inner life—sight, hearing, smell, taste, touch—and we can know without knowing how we know. When you do Reiki on someone at the table, information may be presented to you in the flow of the energy that you perceive with one or more of these inwardly focused senses. It may be fleeting or fragmentary, and it may not seem to make any sense—in the way of dreams.

"If it seems appropriate to share your intuitive impression with the client, describe it to him or her. Ask the client what your description suggests. Don't impose an interpretation. Allow the client to identify the issue being raised, the emotions that are to be explored, the ideas that are to be reconsidered and released. Allow the client to claim the deeper healing that intuitive Reiki can make possible."

"How can we tell what impressions are appropriate to share?" one student asks shyly. "Or maybe that's not the right question. Maybe I should ask instead what kinds of impressions are inappropriate to share?"

"Those are both good questions. First of all, understand that intuitive impressions arise in our minds as we do Reiki to assist in bringing healing. When we dream, the subconscious mind won't release anything to consciousness that is not ready to be healed on some level. So it is with Reiki: when we treat a client, it is as if we dream the client's dream. The intuitive impressions we receive present issues that are ready to be healed by the client on some level.

"However, the client may or may not be open to discussing these issues. For example, if I am treating a new client who is experiencing Reiki for the first time, unless I feel strongly prompted to do so, I will not share any intuitive impressions that come up. I will let them go, without comment.

"If I am treating a regular client, who is familiar with the depth of healing that Reiki can provide, I am likely to ask at the beginning of the treatment, 'Would you like me to tell you about any intuitive impressions that come into my mind during or after the treatment?' Then I will honor the client's request, simply describing what my perceptions are as I go along, or summarizing them, as well as I can remember, at the treatment's end.

"If I am treating another practitioner who is comfortable with intuitive Reiki, I will ask permission to describe whatever impressions arise as soon as they occur, for this encourages a flow of information. This is good practice for me and often a great help to the client."

I pause, considering what I am about to say. "There are times when I do not share intuitive impressions, because it seems inappropriate to do so. For example, if I am working on a cancer patient, and I have an impression that the disease has spread, I will remind myself that I may be receiving an impression about a future possibility, rather than something that has already occurred. Since I am not a doctor I cannot, by law, diagnose, prescribe, or make a prognosis. What I can do is say to the client that I have noticed that there is an intense flow of energy in my hands over an area where I did not expect it to occur. Although that might be due to the acceleration of some perfectly normal bodily function—say, digestion—perhaps it would be wise to let the doctor know and ask for additional tests.

"Or, if I am not comfortable mentioning my impression to the client, I might simply go to Spirit in prayer as I do the treatment and ask for guidance for myself: am I being given this impression so that I will be encouraged to do more Reiki on this client? Often the answer is yes. Then I find a way to treat the client with Reiki on a more regular basis."

The students look somber at this news.

"But I must say that this dilemma occurs very rarely. Usually my impressions are much more commonplace. I see a lot of glasses and pitchers of water, and oranges and bananas. So I describe the image to my clients and ask a question: 'Does this mean anything to you?' Or, if I feel a bit more confident about the reason this image is being presented, I may frame a suggestion: 'Are you getting enough water? Do you think you might need more vitamin C?' Sometimes the person says yes, and sometimes no. What I have found is that it is always best to let the client interpret any impressions that arise for him- or herself.

"Ready to go to the table?"

"Can we take a break first?" The students rise, stretch, yawn. A few step out on the deck for fresh air and a view of blue sky, green grass, and people strolling through the village in the distance.

With Reiki practice as their foundation, I know that, in time, the students will understand that intuition connects us to Source. Intuition teaches us, guards us, and guides us. Intuition gives us "spiritual perception," according to philosophers of old (*Oxford English Dictionary*). We simply need to be willing to accept and use the gift.

INTUITIVE REIKI IN ADVANCED PRACTICE: HANDS-ON

By the time that Reiki practitioners become interested in going on to the advanced course, they have usually had the opportunity to treat at least a few other people besides themselves. They have learned that they can call on the Reiki energy for healing in moments of crisis and periods of calm, and it will flow through their hands to answer the need for healing. They have learned to recognize a wider array of hand sensations as indicative of the flow of Reiki. They have discovered the importance of patience as they wait at the start of a treatment for the energy to begin to flow, and as they wait, during the treatment, with hands in position, through a cycle of the energy for a shift—the signal that they may move their hands to the next position. Finally—and most important—they have learned that Reiki works: it relaxes, relieves pain, accelerates healing, and much more; and they have experienced for themselves these healing benefits, as both client and practitioner.

These experiences are transforming. Practitioners become more confident of their ability to do Reiki—and hope for even greater healing awakens within them. They are ready to go forward with the study of Reiki, to receive additional attunements, and to open up to the extraordinary possibilities for healing that the advanced course presents: offering Reiki to those who are familiar and well-loved—and to those who are unknown—across any geographic distance and across time.

While there are variations in the attunements used, and in the symbols and methods taught in the advanced course, even among the traditional Western lineages, Reiki Masters are generally required to teach their students the use of the first two symbols in hands-on healing. I pass on to my students the use of the first symbol—the power symbol—to call for an increase in Reiki energy in any area of the client's body over which it is physically drawn or visualized by the practitioner. I also pass on to my students the optional use of the second symbol—the mental-emotional healing symbol—at the client's head, physically drawn, always in combination with the first symbol, in the sequence #1–2–1. This sequence of symbols is drawn in the energy field over the client's crown, with the first symbol being gently tapped down on the final stroke each time that it is drawn in the sequence, so that Reiki energy is directed into the eyes; the second symbol is not tapped down but instead floats in the energy field, so that it can best support mental and emotional healing.

In my lineage, however, practitioners are taught that the second symbol has another use. My teacher for Reiki I and II, Reverend Beth Gray, had worked as a professional clairvoyant before learning Reiki to the Reiki Master level from Hawayo Takata. Perhaps for this reason, Beth taught us the use of the second symbol at the client's head not only as the mental-emotional healing symbol, but also as the "talking symbol." When drawn in the sequence #1–2–1, preceded and followed by the first symbol, a safe, protected channel for intuitive Reiki communication is created between client and practitioner. (The second symbol was never to be drawn alone and never to be drawn anywhere but in the energy field over the head.)

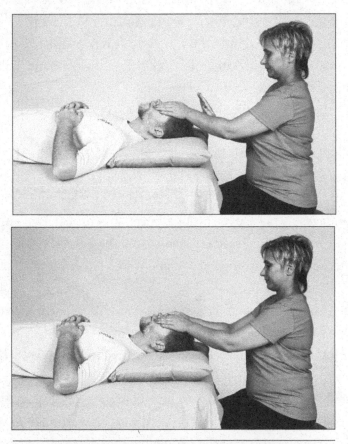

Draw symbols at the head of a client to call for increased Reiki energy and to facilitate intuitive dialogue that can continue through the rest of the treatment.

Of course, many of us still had doubts about our intuitive abilities, even though we were now experienced Reiki practitioners. To allay our concerns, Beth gave us a simple method to try: as we sat at the client's head, after drawing the symbol sequence #1–2–1, we could engage the client in a silent conversation (which she demonstrated for us by speaking out loud). The conversation began with a friendly greeting from the practitioner and a polite inquiry after the client's health, then continued with other questions that helped to identify the client's specific concerns. Finally, the practitioner was to thank the client for providing helpful information and for being present to receive the Reiki treatment. Even in a silent conversation, she told us, it is important to be polite.

When I teach Reiki II students now, I demonstrate the method in the same way that Beth did, saying out loud the words that I normally say in the silence of my mind, so that my students can follow my half of the dialogue. I also describe aloud any impressions that occur in response.

At a recent Reiki II class I taught, this is what occurred.

With my hands placed in position over the eyes of Lauren Bissett, a Reiki II student who had come to assist, I closed my eyes and spoke aloud: "Hello, Lauren. This is Amy. How are you feeling today?" Within a moment or two I saw an image of Lauren, dressed in the black jeans and leotard she wore that day, with protective bandages in place over healing burn scars on her face and arms (the injury that had brought her to Reiki several months before). This Lauren, that I saw with my inner eye, grinned at me and said, "I'm really glad to be here. I really need the Reiki."

I described this impression aloud. I felt Lauren's face crinkle into a smile under my hands.

Next, I asked her, "Lauren, is there any particular area of your body that is in need of healing today?" Immediately I saw her lungs, which looked pink and healthy to me. Nevertheless, I reported this impression aloud.

"Are there any other areas of your body that are in particular need of Reiki?" I asked. I saw an image of her as she was before me, stretched out on the bodywork table. My attention was directed to the inside of her knees. I described this image aloud and went on.

"Are there any issues that concern you at this time that are affecting your health?" I saw an image of Lauren holding a single stalk of celery in her hands, almost as if she were holding a flute. She looked down at the celery with great seriousness. "Hunh!" I said aloud. "I see you holding a stalk of celery." Then I gave in to the temptation to speculate about the image's meaning: "Do you like celery? Do you eat a lot of it? Could you need more fiber in your diet?"

Under my hands I could hear her suppress a chuckle. I knew that she would explain what this image meant to her at the end of the practice session.

I continued our conversation, reporting aloud my questions and impressions. I described a kitchen towel, bright, cheerful, with a printed border of fruit, in a 1950s retro design. I told Lauren that I had the feeling she liked nursing school, thought it was hard, and that she missed her painting. Then I saw another image of her standing upright, looking down skeptically at a little yapping dog—not the beagle I knew she had as pet. The dog was white and it was circling around her ankles. I described this image to her as well. Finally she smiled at me and said, "That's it! That's enough conversation for today." I thanked her for being willing to be the client on the table for this demonstration of intuitive Reiki, then I opened my eyes and lifted my hands away from her head. (With a regular client I would normally conduct this dialogue in silence, and then continue the hands-on treatment through all the positions on the head and the back and any extra positions requested by the client; then, if the client expressed interest, I would describe the impressions I had received to the client for comment.)

Lauren sat up on the bodywork table and grinned at me. "That was amazing!" she said. "Of course, I'm glad to be here. Then right away you saw my lungs." She rolled her eyes. "I wasn't sure whether or not I should tell you, but since I started nursing school this fall, I've started smoking again. Not a lot—just a couple cigarettes here and there. But I quit when I had my accident, and since I've started up again I've been concerned about my lungs."

I reassured her that I wasn't into making judgments, and told her I would be happy to put her on my distant-healing list. She nodded with relief. "And the celery! No, I don't eat a lot of it, but I've been thinking about it a lot, wondering if I should give it up altogether. We've been reading about it in one of my nursing textbooks. It's so hard to digest that I'm not sure that I even want to eat it."

I thought about the image I had seen. She had indeed been studying celery. It would have been better if I had simply described the image to her in more detail rather than trying to speculate about its meaning in my questions to her—but I, too, am still learning! I felt grateful for another lesson from the Reiki energy.

"And what about that area of your knees? Is anything going on there?" I asked.

"Well, yes. Since starting nursing school I'm sitting a lot, crossing my legs at my desk. My knees are bothering me more. They ache.

"And the kitchen towel reminded me of the apartment I just left. I spent so much time in my kitchen. It was the most comfortable room in the house.

"And that dog is my parents' dog. Since I've moved back home with them while I attend nursing school, that dog is around me all the time. He acts like he wants to be picked up, but if I do pick him up, he bites!

"I am glad that I've started nursing school, though. It feels like I've made the right decision. It's hard work, but I miss sleeping!" She laughed. "And I miss my painting. I packed up all my art supplies in August so that I would concentrate on my studies."

"So that treatment was helpful to you?" I asked.

"Yes, especially the message to give Reiki to my lungs and knees. The rest just brought to the surface a lot of things that I've been thinking about."

I smiled in appreciation. "Thank you, Lauren," I said.

"Any time! I can always use the Reiki," she said, and stepped down from the table.

My Reiki II students wanted to know if impressions always flowed that easily. "No, sometimes you don't receive any at all—and that's fine," I said, "because the client is still receiving healing on all levels. Sometimes there isn't a steady flow of images—just an image or two during the course of the whole treatment—and it might occur at any point during the course of the treatment, not just when you are treating the client's head. Occasionally you will have a client like this one, where impressions just keep coming, one right after the other.

"You can encourage that flow by pairing up with another Reiki II practitioner to exchange treatments and practice this method. Ask your partner's permission to 'blurt out' any impressions that arise, as soon as they do so. Have your partner withhold comment until there seem to be no more impressions or you receive a clear message that your inner 'conversation' is over. Then ask for feedback, impression by impression. This the best way that I know to practice this method and to learn to trust the Reiki energy to support you both." I look around at the circle of students, their faces alight with the Reiki energy, their eyes intensely focused.

"Will we get to practice this now with a partner in class?"

I nod. "Yes, we will practice. That's just what we're here to do."

INTUITIVE REIKI IN ADVANCED PRACTICE: DISTANT HEALING

Do intuitive impressions flow as readily when a practitioner does distant healing? Just as with a client treated with hands on, sometimes no intuitive impressions are forthcoming, and this does not indicate any kind of failure on the practitioner's part. (Beth Gray reminded her Reiki II students, in my class and in subsequent classes where I assisted, that not every client is a "Chatty Kathy.") Just as in daily life, we can have clients who are, by nature, quiet and reserved; we can also have clients who, for whatever reason, decide not to "pick up the phone"—to respond to the practitioner's silent invitation to dialogue through intuitive Reiki. While engaging in this dialogue can offer a dimension of mental and emotional healing comparable to that provided by a long talk with a sympathetic friend or a session with a therapist, not every client will choose to enter into it. It is optional, offered by the practitioner, and accepted or declined by the client using free will.

(It is important to note that the practitioner, too, has free will and may choose not to engage in this dialogue, but simply to use the symbols with the intention of enhancing the quality of Reiki healing on all levels. Why might the practitioner decide not to offer this intuitive dialogue in support of healing? Perhaps the practitioner feels a need for mental peace and quiet; or perhaps the practitioner is preoccupied with a personal issue or task and wants to think it through while giving the client a Reiki treatment. While most practitioners enjoy giving their complete attention to the flow of the Reiki energy and the client during a Reiki

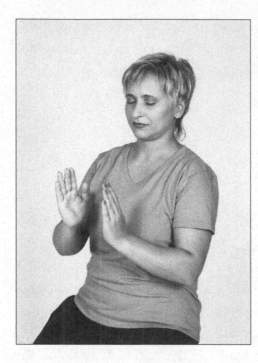

Working at the heart level is comfortable for distant healing.

treatment, there is no requirement—no obligation—that the practitioner do so. Whether or not the practitioner's mind wanders, the Reiki energy still flows and accomplishes its work of healing.)

If it is for the highest good, when the practitioner offers distant healing, the client will accept. If it is also for the highest good, whether or not the practitioner invites the client to engage in an intuitive dialogue, the client may send intuitive impressions. If the practitioner is open to receiving these impressions and willing to record them—with pen and paper or with a tape recorder—during or immediately after the distant-healing session, then this record can provide an additional level of information for the client to consider and use to deepen mental and emotional healing.

Reiki enhances intuition for all practitioners, both traditional and non-traditional, no matter what hand positions or distant-healing methods the practitioners have been taught to use. Whether you have been taught to use a photograph, a proxy, or thought form to connect with your client when you do distant healing, you can ask Spirit—or the Reiki energy itself—to help you to be open to receiving intuitive impressions as you do distant healing. Some distant-healing methods enable you to treat your client in much the same way you would at a bodywork table, using a sequence of hand positions to complete a full treatment. You may discover that, in addition to the sensations of energy that you note in each hand position, you are now aware of images, words, scents, "knowings," that have nothing to do with you, and that you think may or may not have something to do with the client. If so, note them down during or after the treatment. If, on the other hand, you employ a distant-healing method that treats the whole client at once, you may notice that, as you listen closely to the energy in your hands and note specific areas of intensity, other impressions come as well. Note them down during or after the treatment.

If you are treating a client with distant healing who is personally known to you (rather than someone unknown but in need, such as a head of state confronted with a crisis or a group of people affected by a disaster), you may want to consider sharing your impressions. If you do not know the client well or believe the client to be unfamiliar with Reiki, it is probably wisest to keep your notes on the distant-healing session and any impressions you have received to yourself. If you do know the client well and you think that, by sharing your impressions, you may be able to do some good, by all means call or write that individual or arrange a meeting in person. Describe your impressions, and then turn over the process of interpreting them to the client. Remind the client that your impressions, like imagery in dreams, may suggest issues in need of healing, may offer comfort, or may provide validation for a course already chosen.

If you are working on another Reiki practitioner, especially one who has expressed an interest in receiving news of any intuitive impressions received, describe as fully and accurately as you can whatever has come into your mind during the distant-healing session and allow your client to claim the right to interpret these impressions for him- or herself. Take advantage of the opportunity to dialogue about the impressions. Let your practitioner-client ask questions about the impressions to help you recall the subtle details and the nuances of feeling associated with them. This practice will help you become more proficient in relaying impressions accurately; it will also help you and your fellow practitioner-client understand the value of interpretation—the deliberate effort to understand what arises out of the dreamlike communication of intuitive Reiki.

Through interpretation, the client can identify mental and emotional issues in need of healing and begin to understand them in their complexity, to forgive them, and to let them go.

SUGGESTIONS FOR PRACTITIONERS

In a traditionally taught Reiki class we are taught to notice the hand sensations that indicate the energy's flow, often within the span of a single day or weekend. Repeated Reiki attunements, given at intervals during the class, support this remarkably rapid transformation in perception. Once in a while a student still feels uncertain of these hand sensations at the close of the class, yet with regular client practice this student, too, soon develops this ability. Regular practice, in fact, makes it possible for all practitioners to perceive subtle changes in the flow of Reiki energy and to continually refine this perception.

Although many students come to a Reiki class feeling uncertain of their ability to learn Reiki—some say, "I didn't do well in school"; others say, "I'm not very coordinated"; others harbor reservations or feel self-doubt—all are able to learn to sense the energy flow to bring healing and to learn to use this ability quickly and well. Compared to the slow progress a baby makes learning to take those first steps, most Reiki practitioners' progress in learning to perceive the flow of energy is so accelerated that it might be compared to moving at the speed of light, and without a single fall.

Part of the reason for this ease in learning is that the ability to bring healing through touch is natural to every human being, and Reiki enhances that natural ability. Another reason may be that many of those who learn Reiki are highly motivated: they come with the intention of learning Reiki so that they may help loved ones who are in need of healing. Whatever the reasons, practitioners around the world generally do find it easy to learn to listen to the flow of Reiki energy in their hands and to be guided by that flow to complete treatment after treatment.

Every human being also possesses a natural ability to be guided by intuition, which Reiki enhances as well. Yet many people who learn Reiki come to class believing they have little or no intuitive ability; they may also doubt the value of intuition or fear their own perceptions. Gently, over time, Reiki will heal these misconceptions and allay such doubts and fears. Be willing to approach the task of learning intuitive Reiki with patience and love, a commitment to service, and a beginner's mind. You will find that conceptual barriers and limitations fall away. The Reiki energy itself supports this spiritual pathwork.

NOW YOU

Partner with another Reiki practitioner who is interested in becoming proficient in intuitive Reiki. Set up a regular schedule—once a week or every other week—to practice on one another at a bodywork table.

As the practitioner, ask Spirit to help you to be open to receiving intuitive impressions in support of your client's healing throughout the treatment. Simply ask, be open, and relax into the flow of the Reiki energy. Let go of expectations and attachment to outcomes. Let even your mind relax. Enjoy the healing you and your client are both receiving.

As your client prefers, share any impressions that come into your mind during the treatment either as soon as they occur or at the conclusion of the treatment. Just describe. Do not interpret. Ask your client, "Does this impression mean anything to you?" or "Do you understand what this impression is about?"

If your client does understand the impression and chooses to discuss it with you, wonderful. If not, be at peace with your client's decision. If your client doesn't understand an impression, allow yourself—and encourage your client—to be at peace with that as well.

(As a practitioner you will be learning how to sort out your own idle thoughts and projections of your concerns for your client from any intuitive impressions that come. In addition, because the Reiki energy is Spirit-guided energy and Spirit is all-knowing and all-present throughout time, intuitive impressions may occur that refer to the distant past or the near future. This means that sometimes, even when the impressions you receive are accurate, your client may not be immediately able to identify or understand them. Ask your client to follow up the treatment with a phone call if reflection sparks memory or something happens shortly after the treatment that helps to make sense of an impression.)

If you and your Reiki practitioner partner are both advanced practitioners, I urge you to exchange hands-on Reiki treatments, inviting intuition to assist in the healing, until you both begin to feel more comfortable with the process. When you do, you may want to try the intuitive Reiki method described in this chapter, inviting your client to "talk" to you through the protected channel established by the Reiki energy. For the sake of practice, if your partner is willing, simply describe whatever impressions come, without interpretation or judgment, as they occur during the course of treatment. Then ask for your partner's comments. You will both learn a lot from this process. When you feel comfortable and confident using this method in practice with a Reiki practitioner friend, you may decide that you want to offer it to regular clients.

Be willing to be patient with the process of learning intuitive Reiki and with yourself. Reiki is simple, and in time the flow of the energy will offer you intuitive impressions like shells cast up on the beach by gentle waves, whether you are eager to become more intuitive or not.

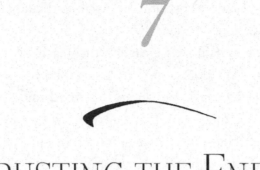

TRUSTING THE ENERGY

As children we learn to walk only by being willing to try to stand and risk a fall. We take a single step, and another, then totter over, having lost our balance. We do this again and again and again—countless times—until finally we are able to stand without falling, to walk forward and cross a room into the arms of someone we love. Soon we are able to walk without even that encouragement, propelled by our desire to explore our environment and to test our new ability. Then we begin to "stretch our legs" in play: we learn to skip, hop, jump, leap, run, dance. Do we fall sometimes? Yes. Does that prevent us from getting up, dusting ourselves off, and trying again? No, not at all. We are beginners: we want to learn, and we accept that learning is a process. We do what is necessary to learn: we accept ourselves, just as we are, and we learn from our successes and our mistakes.

As adults, most of us approach learning a new skill with some trepidation. We may worry about feeling awkward or uncoordinated, being a slow learner, or failing altogether. While these concerns may seem justifiable at the outset, we must set them aside if we are to succeed. One of the reasons that babies are so successful in learning to walk is that they do not evaluate their own efforts critically. They do not sit on the floor after a bad fall and think, "I was really off balance when I took that last step. I'm just so uncoordinated!" They may cry when they fall, because it hurts or because they were startled, but they don't stop themselves from trying again.

Jesus Christ, one of humankind's great spiritual teachers, told his disciples that in order to enter the kingdom of heaven it is helpful to become like a little child. This is wise advice for anyone who wants to advance as a soul. When you are attempting to learn any spiritual skill, be willing to practice it without self-criticism or self-judgment, for these create a sense of struggle that is self-defeating. Be willing to approach learning to meditate, to do yoga, to do Reiki—including intuitive Reiki—with a beginner's mind. Without attachment to a preimposed concept of self as "a slow learner" or "a quick study," without expectation of results on a particular timetable, you will discover that you can enjoy the process of learning to do intuitive Reiki in your own unique way. The Reiki energy—and life itself—will offer you the perfect lesson plan to support your evolution as a soul as you continue on your spiritual journey.

APPRECIATE THE GUIDANCE YOU RECEIVE

Coming to value the intuitive impressions I received as I did Reiki took years. My self-doubts were a strong force during my early practice. For example, when I first began to do Reiki hands-on healing in March 1987, I received few impressions, but one kind of impression that recurred was a glimpse inside the area of the body under my hands, as if my client's skin was transparent. Six months later, after my Reiki II training, I began to see these images of my client's inner organs even more frequently, whether I was working hands-on or sending distant healing. These impressions didn't have much meaning to me, because I had no training in human anatomy or physiology. I couldn't make sense of what I was seeing. Because I did not value these impressions they eventually stopped, to be replaced by others that were more understandable to me.

In retrospect I realize that I was being given a wonderful tool for work as a medical intuitive. At the time, however, my career interests lay elsewhere. I do believe that if I had enrolled in a course on human anatomy or I had begun to do some studying on my own, these impressions would have continued and would be of great value today in my Reiki practice. For those who are already working as nurses, doctors, occupational or physical therapists, or studying to enter one of these professions, understand that Reiki can present such impressions to you—and value them. Your appreciation and gratitude will open your inner senses to receive more.

ALLOW REIKI TO CENTER YOU

Because I lived in Philadelphia when I learned Reiki, an hour or so away from the rest of my family, I looked forward to taking the advanced course so that I could send them healing. However, I was dismayed to discover that I was much more likely to see my worries and fears projected before my inner eye, like a horror movie playing in a darkened theater, than I was to receive any accurate intuitive information. Eventually I realized that the complexity of my feelings for them—concern, sometimes coupled with frustration or even suppressed anger, all overlaying a strong foundation of love—often caused me to imagine the worst. If, for example, my mother had mentioned having an upset stomach after supper, I would find myself picturing her undergoing surgery for a blockage as I sent her distant healing.

This upset me terribly. I felt guilt-ridden at the negativity of my thoughts and fearful that I might somehow have sent them to her, along with healing energy. Would she know? Would she be hurt by them? Would she choose to manifest my most dreaded fears concerning her? Of course, if there were any valid intuitive impressions I might have received, these were obscured altogether by the nightmares created by my imagination.

For a few months I stopped sending Reiki to anyone I loved. It seemed too risky! I intended no harm, but I seemed to have little control over my fears of injury or loss of a family member or dear friend. In time, as I continued to work on others with whom I had less emotional involvement, I found that it was quite possible to send Reiki and receive a variety of impressions, some having to do with the client, some having to do with myself, and some that seemed to be unwanted stray thoughts or projections of my fears. The less attention I gave to such thoughts the more quickly they disappeared. I also discovered that the calmer I felt as I began to send Reiki, the more open and receptive I was to the intuitive impressions from the client and the better able to describe them to the client for interpretation. Other impressions that had a practical value I would consider as possible guidance for myself.

The most receptive state I could manage was a gently contemplative one: the more focused my awareness on the Reiki energy flowing through my hands, the more my mind and emotions quieted and my body relaxed. The flow of Reiki energy through me before it overflowed my hands to heal the client centered me and healed me as well. Often, as I felt the Reiki energy coming in through the crown of my head and flowing downward into my core and then radiating outward to my client, I watched with my eyes closed as the inner light of Spirit seemed to dance: swirls of royal purple, waves of healing greens, circles of golden fire, lightning strikes of white. In this meditative space, healing occurred quickly, effortlessly—and the healing was not only for the client, but also for me.

In time, as I became more whole and less inclined to worry, doubt, and fear, I began again to send Reiki to my mother, father, brother, and other family members. By now I knew from experience that my anxious thoughts are not transmitted to my clients; only the healing energy of Reiki, riding on waves of Spirit's unconditional love, reaches them. My anxiety was itself treated by Spirit as something that needed healing in me. The sooner I accepted that healing, the sooner I felt the gentle rush of Reiki into my hands and the more effective I could be in treating the client.

Now, before I begin distant healing, I take time to do a technique that is done by Japanese Reiki practitioners and masters to clear the aura: Kenyoko-ho or dry brushing (see chapter 13 for complete, step-by-step instructions). With a few quick strokes of my hands across my heart and down my arms, I clear away any undesirable thoughts and negative feelings I have experienced or been exposed to during the day, just as if I were sweeping away sticky cobwebs. Then I bring my hands together at the heart level, palm to palm, to establish my connection to the energy. (This hand position, which Westerners associate with prayer, the Japanese call *gassho* and use to begin and end meditation.) Finally, I recite the

Reiki principles with thoughtfulness and care. These three small ritual acts go far to calm and center me, so that I may be filled quickly to overflowing with Reiki to be sent on its way to my clients, and my mind may be like a calm, clear lake in which impressions of my client's inner landscape are gently and beautifully reflected.

TRUST REIKI TO TEACH YOU

One of my first lessons from the Reiki energy put me into a near panic. As an apartment dweller, I missed having a pet. So I was pleased when a cat, who had been abandoned by her owner, had four kittens in the crawl space under the apartment building next to me. I began setting out dry cat food and water in an empty garage behind the building for this hungry brood. After a few weeks of this ritual, the mother cat made friends with me, rubbing against my legs and allowing me to pet her. The kittens didn't want to get close.

One day I noticed—from a safe distance—that two of the kittens had eye infections. All I could do was to send Reiki distant healing, and apparently, over the course of a few days, this was enough to clear up the infections. After this the kittens became bolder and friendlier, although they still had no interest in sniffing my hands.

Over the course of a couple of months the kittens grew and became more playful. One day, with the mother cat leading the way, they followed me upstairs to my second-floor apartment. I left the door open so that they would not feel trapped, and after several minutes of exploring they retreated down the stairs. Over the next two or three weeks they made several visits like this, always returning to their dirty crawl space.

One evening in early fall, when the kittens were about four months old, I came home from work to discover two of them on my porch step, side by side, one holding up his paw. They were waiting for me! I opened the door and the two of them bounded up the stairs. This time, knowing one of them was injured, I shut the door behind them. When I finally got close enough to the little black and white kitten to see what was wrong, I was horrified to discover that he had sheared off a toe pad. There was no blood, just an unsupported claw.

I called a veterinary hospital immediately, described the cat's injury, and then was interviewed so the hospital could set up a file.

"What is the name of the cat?" the receptionist asked.

"He doesn't have a name."

"Who is the owner?"

"The cat is an alley cat, a stray."

"Has the cat had a rabies shot?"

"No, I'm certain he hasn't. The cat lives in a crawl space under the building next to me. He's never had shots."

"Do you know how he received this injury?"

"I have no idea."

"If you bring the cat in, under Pennsylvania state law we will be required to put the animal to sleep or to quarantine it for six months."

"What? Could you repeat that, please?" I was stunned.

Knowing that I could not afford to pay for six months of boarding this kitten, I set down the receiver. I looked up the number of another veterinary hospital and called. I received the same answers. I tried yet another veterinary hospital and was told the same dismaying facts again. This receptionist, at least, was sympathetic to my desire to care for a stray. She told me that if I could catch the cat, I should clean the injury and use a bit of antibiotic ointment on it. In all likelihood the cat would lick the ointment off, but it was worth trying.

When I finally got off the phone I sat, thinking, for a long time. What could I really do? The only healing I could truly offer was Reiki. Yet the injury seemed so serious. Would Reiki be enough?

I called a practitioner friend. "Listen, I have one of those kittens here that I mentioned to you, and he's injured. Could you come over and have a look at him, so that you can send some distant healing, too?"

Then I tried to catch the cat, who clearly preferred to hide under chairs and behind the couch. Eventually I did catch him. I held him while he fought me, so that I could clean the injury and apply ointment. I left the apartment briefly to get a litter box and other supplies at a grocery store. When I returned, I began to send Reiki to the cat.

"You need a name," I told him, as he huddled in a corner, as far away from me as he could get. Because of the black spot on the top of his head, he made me think of the Dr. Seuss book *The Cat in the Hat*. So I named him Seuss, and treated him, with the help of my friend, to many hours of Reiki over the next few days.

Seuss's injury healed well, and eventually became hidden under white fur. I adopted Seuss and his family long before they adopted me. He sleeps now, content, curled into a warm ball, on a chair just a few feet away from me.

This Reiki lesson pushed me to the limit of my ability and past my skepticism. When these two cats turned up on my doorstep, they knew instinctively—or intuitively—that Reiki energy could help heal this injury. I didn't. I learned from their trust in the energy to trust it myself more completely.

ASK FOR CLARIFICATION

Like many Reiki practitioners trained in this traditional lineage to do intuitive Reiki, I doubted the validity of the impressions I received at first. Sometimes I felt as if I was trying too hard, and at other times I felt as though I wasn't trying hard enough. It took a couple of years for me to understand the importance of letting go of this sense of struggle. As I began to relax and trust the Reiki energy more and more, I also began to feel comfortable with speaking out—or noting down—the impressions I received as they came to me, without judgment.

However, there were more lessons to be learned. One evening I had a dinner date. When my friend did not arrive on time, I began to worry. When he was half an hour late I decided to send distant healing and to ask for impressions concerning his welfare. I connected to him through the energy and immediately asked, "Have you been in an accident?"

I saw an image of his head hitting the windshield of his car, shattering the glass. I saw the blood in his hair and then darkness. My heart began to pound in fear, as I became even more worried about him.

About five minutes later he knocked on the door, and I opened it to him. He was fine. I asked, "Have you been in an accident?"

He answered flatly, as if this were not a strange question, "Yes, I was in an accident about six months ago. My head hit the windshield and broke the glass. I was in the hospital for three days with a concussion." As I let this register I asked why he was so late, and he explained that he had been delayed by heavy traffic.

In the days that followed this experience, I thought about how my question to him during distant healing had been a projection of my worry. Perhaps if I stayed calm, I reasoned, I would be less likely to see my own nightmares played out on that mental screen. It seemed I needed to remind myself of the Reiki principles, especially, "Just for today, do not worry," before I sent distant healing. I also understood that the impression I was shown had been accurate in describing an event that had taken place six months earlier. I had forgotten that to Spirit and to the Reiki energy, all time is now. In my anxiety I had neglected to ask, "When is this occurring?" If I had remained calm enough to ask for clarification, I might have spared myself some emotional pain.

PAY ATTENTION TO FEELINGS

To allow the Reiki energy to calm me and relieve any sense of concern I had about my clients before I began to send them distant healing, I took a simple step: I sent Reiki to myself first; sometimes, in addition, I would meditate. In session after session this seemed to smooth the way for more accurate intuitive impressions to occur. Yet there was still another lesson to learn about the importance of what I was feeling.

Over the course of about a year, I developed constant pain in both kidneys. Medical tests showed no infection, although I was given an antibiotic as a preventive. Whenever I sent Reiki to myself, I saw an image of an old-fashioned water faucet with a slow drip. Something about the water faucet felt disturbing to me, but I dismissed this feeling again and again because it didn't match the advice my doctor was giving me: drink more water.

One morning one of the dogs in the house where I was staying had a seizure. The veterinarian diagnosed lead poisoning, probably from drinking water with a high lead content. When the dog was hydrated with fresh, pure water, she recovered quickly. At home we gave her bottled water, and I began to drink it as well.

Within the next few days we had the water that came out of the kitchen faucet tested. It showed high spikes of lead to dangerous levels; the house was old, and the plumbing pipes were lined with lead, which had been leaching into the water. Every morning I had run the faucet to fill the coffee pot and the dog's water dish with that water.

Finally, I understood the message I had been receiving as I did Reiki: there *was* something wrong with the water faucet, and if I had not ignored that feeling, I might have prevented the dog's seizure and my long bout of kidney pain. Within about three days of switching to bottled water my health recovered as well. The importance of paying attention to the feelings associated with an intuitive impression and asking for clarification when I received a confusing impression had been brought home to me in a very personal way.

LEARNING TO TRUST THE PROCESS

The importance of becoming quiet and centered before I began to use intuitive Reiki to send distant healing was brought home to me on several occasions. In my family, we celebrate birthdays without a lot of fanfare: we get together after dinner for birthday cake and ice cream at home, then watch as the birthday honoree opens a few well-chosen presents. On March 3, 1996, we had planned to meet at my brother Mark's house, with his wife and children, at 6 PM to celebrate his thirty-ninth birthday. This would allow everyone ample time to drive home, including my father, who worked in construction and who would need a few extra minutes to shower and change.

As six o'clock approached my mother and I sat down on the couch in the family room to wait for my father. She picked up an old photo album and began paging through it, stopping occasionally to tell me a story about a relative in one of the pictures: my great grandfather who was given a speeding ticket for racing a bicycle across the newly built Brooklyn Bridge; my uncle who broke his arm as a small boy by jumping off a garage roof, pretending an umbrella was a parachute. We had a digital clock on an end table that kept us apprised of the time, and a perfect view of the western sky through a picture window.

As the minutes ticked by we saw the sun slip down closer to the horizon, its cool golden rays backlighting the trees on the wooded slope below, silhouetting the bare branches and tall trunks. Then the more distant woods across the field below seemed to tangle the sun in dark treetops. The sun flashed to the bright orange flare of an ember, then suddenly went out.

It was now close to seven o'clock. My mother suggested that I advise my brother and his family that we would be delayed; my father was still not home, and we had received no word from him.

After the call I settled back down on the couch beside her. She seemed to be studying the photos intently, deliberately keeping her mind off the possible reasons for my father's unexpected delay. Without disturbing her, I reached for a couch pillow, put it on my lap, and connected to my father using Reiki distant healing. As my hands slowly moved through the positions on the pillow, I talked to him silently. Was he alright? Had he been in an accident? Even though I now knew from experience that this could be a leading question, I felt a need to know.

"No," he said. "I haven't been in an accident, but you're not going to believe that after a while—and I could use the Reiki anyway. So please continue."

I was stumped. I asked for clarification and had only an impression of lots of headlights, not moving, in increasing darkness. I didn't know what to make of it, but I continued sending Reiki as he had requested, until my mother and I left the house at 7:15 to go to my brother's house.

My brother and sister-in-law and their three children, my mother and I, and a couple of my brother's friends and their wives enjoyed an informal dinner in the kitchen before we moved into the living room for my brother to open his gifts. Although we talked and laughed, we were not as lighthearted as we pretended to be. All the adults were being quite careful not to show the anxiety we felt. None of us wanted to alarm the children.

At about 9:30 my sister-in-law made the children say good night to us all and sent them up to bed. My mother and I said good night as well, collected our coats, and drove to my parents' home, which was just a few minutes away. Once we got in the door we began to talk about whether or not we should start calling local hospital emergency rooms that would have been along my father's route home. We decided to continue to wait.

Finally, around ten o'clock, we heard my father's truck in the driveway. When he opened the door into the kitchen, we were both there to greet him, wanting to know by the evidence of our eyes that he was safe and unharmed. And so he was: he still wore his work clothes, and except for being tired and sweaty, he seemed fine.

He told us what had delayed him right away. As he was driving north on Route 309, one of the major arteries out of Philadelphia into the northern suburbs, a hazardous waste truck had jack-knifed in the middle of an intersection and spilled its contents all over the road. In all four directions approaching the intersection, all traffic had been stopped, except for emergency vehicles, until the spill could be completely cleared away. This process had taken close to four hours. He was sure, he said, that there were many other people just like him, only getting home now—at ten o'clock at night—from their work day.

He called my brother to apologize for missing the birthday celebration and for causing unneeded worry, got a sandwich for himself, and then retired to take a shower and go to bed.

I went home, but not to bed. I had too much on my mind to sleep. I needed to think! When my father told me, through the Reiki connection, that he had not been in an accident, but that after a while I would not believe him, he was right. With each hour that he was delayed, it had become more difficult not to dwell on tragic possibilities.

On balance, though, his comment had also provided some reassurance. In those moments when I had been able to bring myself to trust the accuracy of the impression and accept his statement at face value, I had relaxed and breathed more easily. Initially, I did not find it difficult to trust that he was safe, but as it got later, this became much harder to do. To fight back my fear I had reminded myself of the second Reiki principle: "Just for today, do not worry." This was the life preserver I had gripped as the stormy sea of my emotions threatened to sweep over me again and again.

Most practitioners learn to trust the constancy of Reiki's healing qualities over time, through experience. In the early years of practice this may mean understanding that Reiki consistently accelerates healing or always relieves pain; later on, as intuitive impressions come more often, time is needed to learn to trust their accuracy.

Yet every Reiki practitioner can use the Reiki principles from day one to find that peaceful center within and feel safe and at home. The Reiki principles define the basic choices we can make each day to claim health and well-being: to remain calm, to project a positive attitude, to be grateful for the gift of life, to strive to do our best and work with integrity, to be kind to everyone we meet. Dr. Usui found the Reiki principles worthy of daily contemplation and meditation. Although they are not given great emphasis in Western Reiki teaching, they, too, have a healing power that should never be underestimated; consideration of the Reiki principles enables us to open up to receive greater spiritual guidance and help.

TRUSTING EVEN MORE DEEPLY

Sending Reiki to the planet for peace and healing is so important that I ask every Reiki practitioner I train in distant healing to consider making it a part of daily practice.

When I send Reiki to the planet, I usually start with the remembered images of NASA photographs of Earth from space. Then I feel its roundness and see it slowly turning on its axis as it hangs suspended in the star-studded darkness of the Milky Way. As I focus on the turning world and send healing, sometimes my intuition seems to zoom in like a camera with a telephoto lens. All of a sudden I am looking at an African tribesman cutting down grasses or a deer drinking from a forest stream or a woman in a suit and high heels purposefully striding down a city street. I do not know what I see, but I do assume that whatever comes to my awareness needs healing.

During the summer of 1998, over a period of weeks, each time I sent Reiki to the earth I saw smoke billowing over the Pacific. This seemed odd since I had heard of no earthquakes or volcanoes that might account for the billowing gray clouds that curved around the slowly turning world. Was I imagining this impression? Or could I be glimpsing the effects of some future disaster? I considered these questions but continued to send Reiki, believing on the basis of past experience that the few minutes of time I spent in sending distant healing to the planet would only do good.

Finally a story broke in the news: fires had been raging out of control for weeks on the tiny island of Jakarta in the Pacific. Now the smoke and dust had been blown by ocean air currents as far as the shores of California. The smoke was adding to the smog problems in Los Angeles and other cities along the West Coast. And on the island of Jakarta itself, the few firefighters were exhausted and at the end of their resources. The government had appealed to other nations to send additional crews of trained firefighters to help quench the flames. The story remained front-page news for weeks until finally the flames were extinguished and the island returned, more or less, to normal life. I continued to send Reiki to the planet, now without noticing smoke trails over the Pacific.

This experience was a practical lesson for me in global consciousness. Although I count my contribution to world healing through Reiki as very slight, my intuition, riding the flow of Reiki energy, could sense an enduring need for healing roughly halfway around the world. Even though I doubted these impressions as they continued to appear day after day, week after week, they were finally explained. While I sent energy for world healing, the energy worked to heal me of my world of doubts—and I am better for it: instead of taking on faith the existence of a loving higher power that guides all life on planet Earth, now I know that higher power exists.

SUGGESTIONS FOR PRACTITIONERS

The ability to receive intuitive impressions while doing Reiki, to recognize their value, and to communicate them appropriately to the client has been taught only within a few traditional Western lineages. Yet this ability can be learned by any practitioner who is willing to approach the task with "beginner's mind" and to work with the Reiki energy over time to develop it into a skill that can be used effectively to support Reiki healing.

There are several self-limiting choices a practitioner can make that slow or stop the development of intuitive ability. Simply by choosing not to value intuition the practitioner may stall its development. The practitioner may also choose not to value self (dismissing intuitive impressions as "idle daydreams") or to overvalue self (presenting any intuitive impressions that come with arrogance and false authority) with the same result.

How, then, can a practitioner learn to be more intuitive? Supported by a foundation of experiences with Reiki, even the most hesitant and self-doubting practitioner can learn to set aside negative ego, relax in the flow of the energy, and listen. Listen with the same slightly heightened awareness that is used to listen to hand sensations: peaceful, centered, compassionate, receptive, present. Listen, as experience with the Reiki energy teaches every practitioner to do over time, to the energy flowing not only through the hands but through the whole being. Notice what arises on this flow: a tingling under the fingertips, a gently, coursing current in the back of the head, a soft cascade of warmth over the face, pulsing in the soles of the feet, an arc of golden light against a curtain of purple, seen behind closed eyelids. It is in this relaxed enjoyment of the Reiki energy radiating through one's whole being that intuition arrives.

NOW YOU

The world is in need of healing, on all levels of being, just as we are. One of the blessings of learning Reiki distant healing is that we can incorporate sending Reiki to the world into our daily practice. Some of us may be drawn to focus healing on specific areas of the world: for example, Pakistan in the aftermath of an earthquake, Central America in the wake of hurricane rains and mud slides, the coral reefs that are the habitats for so much ocean life. Others will want to ask for Reiki healing to be sent more broadly, to the biosphere, or to Earth and its energy fields, including the electromagnetic fields and energy grid that stabilize the planet.

If you are an advanced Reiki practitioner, you will already be familiar with a method for sending healing from your Reiki II class. You may already be using this method to send Reiki for world healing. If not, here is a simple way that will work for any advanced practitioner.

1. Raise your hands up in front of you, at the level of your heart, with your palms facing each other and a small space in between.
2. Imagine planet Earth in this space. Name the whole Earth or the part of Earth to which you want to send healing.
3. Offer Reiki, acknowledging free will and higher purpose.
4. Make the Reiki symbols for distant healing in the sequence you were taught. Then return the hand with which you drew the symbols to its original position.
5. Listen to the Reiki energy as it flows between your hands, sending healing.
6. When you feel the flow of energy begin to diminish, bring the treatment to a close with an expression of thanks or a blessing, then break the connection by blowing into the space between your hands, clapping, rubbing your hands together, or bringing them together as if in prayer.

If you are a Reiki practitioner but are not yet trained in distant healing, you will discover that you can use the method described above without the symbols, but with strong, clear intention to bring Reiki healing.

Can you receive intuitive impressions as you send Reiki healing to the world? Yes! As with all Reiki, daily practice will make you feel more comfortable with the process and will continually refine your awareness of subtle energy. As you listen to your hands you may discover that you are also seeing images of the African veldt, of a parrot perched in a tropical rainforest, of a person unknown to you, looking tired and disheveled, traveling in a taxicab through a foreign city. Work with the energy each day—and ask to be open to receiving intuitive impressions as you do. You will do no harm, and your patient practice will bring only healing.

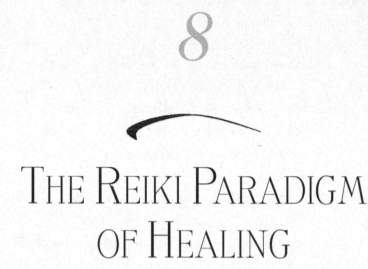

THE REIKI PARADIGM OF HEALING

Reiki is distinguished from many other holistic and allopathic healing methods by the healing benefits that it brings to the practitioner, even as the practitioner is engaged in treating a client. Unlike massage, for example, which requires the massage therapist to use his or her own physical energy to manipulate the client's muscles in order to relieve tension and stimulate improved circulation, Reiki does not use the practitioner's own energy or demand arm strength or endurance. After giving five or six massages in a row, a massage therapist is usually tired and drained, well aware that this has been a hard day's work; at the end of a full day of treating Reiki clients, a practitioner is likely to feel alert, clear-headed, energetically charged, and capable of doing more. After months or years of the repetitive motions required to knead muscle tissue into a relaxed state, massage therapists often develop carpal tunnel syndrome in their wrists and arms. After the same period of time, a Reiki practitioner with a stable of regular clients is likely to feel healthier than ever. (These differences have motivated many massage therapists to learn Reiki and add it their repertoire of holistic healing skills.)

The Reiki practitioner's improved health and well-being may be the result of daily self-treatment, but every client treatment brings healing benefits to the practitioner as well. The Reiki energy flows through the practitioner, relaxing, calming, centering, before it overflows the practitioner's hands, transmitting healing energy to the client. The universal life-force energy that flows into and through the practitioner always brings some healing to the practitioner, even when a client is the intended recipient. In this way Reiki offers the ideal experience of healing: practitioner and client both feel better.

Sometimes, however, it is necessary to consciously set and maintain boundaries in order for the practitioner to receive these healing benefits. While the repeated attunements given during a traditional Reiki class effectively open, stabilize, reinforce, and "seal" from negativity the channel for healing energy created within each practitioner, occasionally an individual who is particularly empathic—sensitive to the pain of others—will express a concern during the class about this unconscious habit. "When I put my hands on my clients," the practitioner will ask, "am I going to feel the ache of their arthritis or the weakness they feel after the flu? Am I going to feel their pain?" For these empathic individuals, who have learned that they have a tendency to take on others' pain through physical proximity or hands-on contact, specific instructions should be provided by the Reiki Master.

Beth Gray recommended to her Reiki I students that any practitioner who registered the client's pain, either in the hands or the physical body, break the connection with the client by removing the hands from wherever they were positioned and shaking them out. Taking this simple step would relieve the practitioner's muscle tension and stiffness. Then the practitioner could resume the same hand position. If pain in the practitioner's hands or body then recurred, it was a clear signal that the practitioner was taking on the client's pain. The way to eliminate it was to say to oneself and to Spirit, clearly and firmly, "This is not my pain. Please have it leave me now." If the pain did not immediately dissipate, the statement was to be repeated until it did.

In retrospect, I realize that this was one of those moments in my Reiki training when the secular and spiritual nature of the information being presented to us was blurred. I did not mind at the time, nor do I now. However, I feel that the technique works even more effectively if the practitioner is aware that Reiki offers us the opportunity to work in complete harmony with Spirit. We can ask Spirit for help, for protection, for guidance, for clarification, for direction at any time during a treatment, and "it shall be given" to us (Matthew 7:7).

While most people who learn Reiki never experience the problem of taking on the client's pain, for those who are sometimes this empathic, at least with family members or friends, I teach the technique that Beth presented in my Reiki I classes. I also invite my students to enlarge on their dialogue with Spirit. If the reason for the client's pain is known, I suggest that the student say, "Thank you, Spirit, for this information, but I am already aware of the client's condition. Please send the pain away now." If the reason for the client's pain is not known, I recommend that the student say instead, "Thank you, Spirit, for this information, but this is not my pain. Please show me in another way and have the pain leave me now." This works—and invites the information to come as an intuitive impression in another form—an image, a word or phrase, a knowing.

For the record, within the Japanese tradition practitioners are not discouraged from registering pain as a momentary hand sensation over *byosen*—diseased areas of the body (for more information about this, please see chapter 13). The impression is considered to have diagnostic value. Since I have learned to practice and teach Reiki in both traditions, I am conscious that the practitioner has some choice—and I choose not to experience unnecessary pain as I do a Reiki treatment on a client. I encourage my students to make the same choice and to enjoy and accept all the healing benefits Reiki has to offer.

SEND AWAY UNNECESSARY PAIN

During one of the very first Reiki classes I taught I had an international group of students: an American couple, a Russian student, and an Israeli man who told me, as soon as he walked in the door, that he had come to America to learn to be a shaman and he was willing to take on the suffering of others in order to relieve their pain.

"Whoa!" I said. "Please understand that shamanism, while an ancient and honorable tradition of healing, is very different from Reiki. When you do Reiki on a client you receive healing, as does the client. You are not meant to take on the client's pain. There's no reason to do so. You don't lessen the client's pain by taking it on. It still needs healing, only now you are the one who needs the healing. Reiki offers something very special: healing for your client and for you."

I reviewed with this student the method of sending away pain, if it occurred. He nodded his understanding and acceptance, and I continued to teach the class over the next two days. During the final practice session I was his client for hands-on treatment. He moved through the hand positions of Basic I (over the front of the torso), listening intently to the energy. When he reached fourth position (the V inside the pelvic cradle), he cried out: "Oh, I feel a sharp, stabbing pain, like a knife, across my knuckles!"

"You don't need to feel that pain," I told him. "It's twenty years old, and I know exactly what caused it—I had surgery there! Send the pain away and ask to receive the information in another way."

He agreed to try and was able to free himself of the sensation of pain in his hand. I trust that, as he has continued to practice, he has had other opportunities to use this technique to refuse pain as an intuitive impression.

Even though I recognize the importance of refusing pain, there were a few years when I willingly accepted a sensation of itchiness in my hands because it helped me to recognize that a client had allergies. Eventually I realized that this discomfort was also a form of pain and not necessary. I could ask to receive the same information—that my client had allergies—in another way, and I needed to trust the Reiki energy to make that information available to me, if it was for the client's highest good.

With a close friend or family member it is more difficult to set this boundary. While treating a friend who was prone to kidney stones, I became aware of the exact location of the large stone she was about to have surgically removed, because I could feel the sharp pain in my own body. I had to break contact, shake out my hands, acknowledge to myself that I already had this information and that the pain was unnecessary, before I could continue and complete the treatment.

The same issue can occur during Reiki distant healing, particularly when a practitioner is not only sending healing but is also receiving intuitive impressions from the client. While most impressions feel neutral, some are emotionally charged. Registering a client's psychic pain can be just as—or even more—unpleasant than registering a client's physical pain. Again, this pain is unnecessary and can be avoided by learning to set boundaries and work with clear intention.

LEVELS OF CONNECTION

In the late 1980s, as I assisted at a Reiki II class, I was particularly drawn to watching one woman during the distant healing practice session. All the students—about two dozen—were seated around conference tables, with their pillows resting on the varnished table surface in front of them. As they sent Reiki to clients unknown to them, except as a face in a photograph and a name, their faces were intent, as if they listened to faraway music. Most had their eyes closed as their hands rested in position, sending Reiki healing energy.

The woman whose face I found most arresting was as quietly focused as any of her classmates, but her face was streaked with tears. As I watched, still more tears glistened at the corners of her eyes and fell. She cried in complete silence, apparently not wanting to disturb the air of deep concentration in the room.

At the close of the treatment time each of the newly trained Reiki II practitioners was invited to share any intuitive impressions received with the class. This helped everyone to become more comfortable with the varied ways in which the information was transmitted from the clients and perceived by the practitioners. This also created a safe space for the practitioner who had requested the distant healing for the relative or friend in the shared photograph to confirm any accurate impressions and make any other appropriate comments. It was reassuring for new Reiki II practitioners to see their classmates struggle to overcome self-doubt, just as they were attempting to overcome their own, and it was wonderful to witness their surprised smiles as, again and again, they were told, "Yes, that's exactly like her," or, "I've heard him use those very words." As each practitioner shared impressions and received some validation, all the practitioners grew in understanding and confidence. The feeling of excitement was almost palpable—

and moved through the group like the lighting of candle after candle, becoming bright flames against the darkness.

In this group, the woman who cried captured everyone's attention early on. She was asked what impressions she had received about her client, an elderly woman. Very seriously, she said, "I felt so much sadness—and all I saw was a dotted field of gray. I asked to be shown the information in another way, but nothing else came . . . just this terrible sadness and that gray. Maybe—maybe I just can't do this."

The teacher did not give the practitioner's self-doubt any reinforcement. "Let's find out more about your client," she said, looking pointedly at the practitioner who had supplied the photograph of the elderly woman. "Perhaps your impressions are more accurate than you realize."

The practitioner who had brought the photo to class nodded. "That's my mother, and she is sad. She's had Alzheimer's disease for years. It's a long time since she's recognized me or anyone else in the family, and she does seem to feel a sense of loss. I think you picked up on her depression at having all of her memories of her family gradually slip away from her. I think now she feels terribly alone and sad. I'm not surprised that the only image she showed you was of a gray field with dots. It makes sense. So much of her mind is gone."

The practitioner who had sent distant healing to the woman with Alzheimer's sighed, relieved that she had been accurate, but distressed for her classmate. "I'm so sorry. It must be so difficult for you to cope with your mother's illness."

"It's one of the reasons I'm here. I'm hoping that by sending her Reiki distant healing, I can reach her and relieve some of her suffering."

They smiled at one another, united in sympathy and spiritual purpose: to act with compassion, to bring healing with kindness. They thanked one another, and the class continued, with a deeper awareness of the power of Reiki.

During the years that followed this class, I often thought about the woman who had cried. In class after class at which I assisted, new Reiki practitioners were reminded not to take on the clients' pain. "It's a piece of information," we were told. "Now you know where your client hurts—but it is not necessary to feel pain in order to receive that information. Send the pain away. Be firm. Ask Spirit to show you this information in another way."

While I did not often pick up my client's pain as I did Reiki hands-on, it happened a few times. On these occasions I followed the recommendation to send the pain away and found prompt relief. I knew the method also had worked well for other Reiki practitioners. But what about emotional, mental, or spiritual pain? This was the question that formed in my mind as I reflected on the practitioner who had cried while sending Reiki distant healing to the woman with Alzheimer's disease. Clearly, she had picked up her client's emotional pain. Was there some way to protect against receiving such distressing emotions? Could such a feeling be refused or avoided altogether by setting clear boundaries, and accurate intuitive impressions still be received?

In the course of a phone conversation, a fellow practitioner made the sensible suggestion to connect to any client who might be in emotional turmoil on a "high self" or soul level. This would surely provide a higher, wiser perspective on whatever circumstances or conditions the client was facing.

Shortly after this advice, I was given a practical reminder to share it with my own Reiki II students. One summer weekend, three women came to my home to take a Reiki II class. After I had attuned and taught them symbols and methods, they practiced, first hands-on at the bodywork tables and then distant healing on a client unknown to them. Each Reiki practitioner had brought a photograph of someone in need of healing.

Now each practitioner exchanged her photograph with another student, providing the name of the person in the photo as well. One of the photos showed an image of a bearded man on a motorcycle. After the practice session, the practitioner who treated this man with distant healing seemed quite upset as she described the many impressions she had received. Struggling to keep her voice steady, she told us that she thought he had a very hard life; she had seen images of a needle going into an arm and speculated that he might have used drugs. He did not seem well, and he did seem to be in a lot of emotional turmoil. She wondered aloud if he were still alive, and if he were, if he might be dying.

The practitioner who had supplied this man's photograph confirmed many of these impressions. Indeed, he had been a drug user in his twenties and had contracted HIV from sharing a needle with a fellow user. Now in his thirties, he had AIDS and was alternately angry and depressed to the point of despair; he might even be suicidal.

As the practitioner who had sent Reiki to this man heard her impressions explained and confirmed, tears of sympathy and sadness for him streaked her cheeks. I realized then that a practitioner has a right and a responsibility to protect himself or herself from emotional, mental, and spiritual pain, as well as from physical pain. It is not necessary to pick up a client's feelings of fear, anger, despair, or confusion.

I shared with these students my friend's recommendation to connect to such troubled clients on a high self or soul level. This safely steps down the intensity of feeling received as intuitive impressions while providing access to the overview of the life plan that is the soul's wisdom.

By specifically requesting to connect to a client—or a group of clients—on a soul level, it even becomes possible to send distant healing to those who are victims of terrible disasters without being overwhelmed. In the aftermath of the terrorist attacks on September 11th, many Reiki practitioners sent healing in this way to the victims, the family and friends who survived them, and to the emergency personnel and volunteers who labored to rescue survivors, recover bodies, and clear the site. This is one of the practical ways in which Reiki is used for world healing.

MAKE NO "PRONOUNCEMENTS OF DOOM"

One evening at a Reikishare, I witnessed a first-time visitor become terribly upset as she placed her hands over a client's chest. She left the table suddenly, and I followed her to see if I could help in any way. Although she had never received any training in how to recognize or relay intuitive impressions received as she did Reiki, she had registered a very strong one. With tears in her eyes she told me, "He's going to have a heart attack." I asked her to sit with me and think about why she might have received this impression.

Could it be to warn the client of a potential health problem, so that he might take steps to prevent it? Yes, she agreed, it could. In her experience, were there any steps she might recommend to the client to help prevent this outcome? Yes, she said, there were several herbal supplements she could suggest that were good for the heart. He has free will, I reminded her. He might indeed take her advice. I suggested that she talk with him, sharing her impression and mentioning these supplements.

She did so. He tried the supplements and found them unpalatable, then visited his doctor to have his cholesterol checked. The doctor prescribed Lipitor, which lowered his cholesterol within a few month's time, altering the sad outcome this woman had foreseen with such surety to a positive one: the client made a decision to have his doctor monitor his heart health. Now, several years later, he remains in good health.

This experience reminded me that there is another kind of boundary in the practitioner-client relationship that must be respected. No practitioner should make predictions about a client's future health, no matter how strong or clear the impressions might seem. First, it is illegal, the province of physicians only, to make a diagnosis and prognosis. Second, the client has free will and may make choices at any time that alter the future. Third, it is manipulative, effectively taking away the client's power to claim complete healing.

Intuitive impressions received by practitioners during a Reiki treatment on a client may suggest future possibilities, but the future is not predetermined. In fact, intuitive Reiki can present future possibilities to the mind of the practitioner as a call for more healing.

It is good practice simply to present any impressions received to the client for interpretation, rather than trying to interpret them yourself. I recommend gently framing the question, "Does this mean anything to you?" This allows the client to come to a conscious awareness of the impression's meaning, either during the Reiki session or in the hours or days that follow.

SUGGESTIONS FOR PRACTITIONERS

Take some time to appreciate how Reiki healing works. Can you think of any other healing modality that offers benefits to the practitioner as well as the client?

What healing have you felt yourself receiving as you treated others? Have you noticed physical tension and pain washing away in the flow of Reiki energy? Have you been aware of your own emotional distress dissolving into Reiki light as a feeling of calm settled over you? Have you realized that your mind was more clear and alert after treating a client than before? Be grateful for the healing you have received whenever you have offered Reiki to a client, as well as for the healing you have received during self-treatment.

NOW YOU

Recall the history of your Reiki client practice. Have you ever noticed pain in your hands above an area of pain in a client's body or registered a client's pain with pain in your own body, at the same location? While this happens only rarely for most practitioners, it can be unsettling when it occurs. Let the memory go, and know that you now have the instruction you need to set a clear boundary between yourself and your client, if and when such a situation recurs. You may want to send Reiki distant healing to yourself back in time to any client session in which you picked up pain as an intuitive impression to help you to free yourself from any anxiety about this issue that you have carried into the present.

Consider the difference between empathy—the ability to feel another's pain—and sympathy—the ability to comfort another who is in pain by understanding and acknowledgment. Consciously recognize that empathy has no real value in Reiki practice. Instead, practice sympathy and kindness.

Finally, have compassion for yourself. Forgive your own mistakes in all areas of your life, and learn from them as best you can. Don't punish yourself by anchoring your identity in the past. Allow Reiki to bring you healing on all levels, and accept that healing. Grow spiritually, and outgrow low self-esteem, diminished self-respect, faltering self-doubt, or worse, self-loathing. Reiki has been called "the energy of unconditional love." Search for self-understanding, forgive your past mistakes, and discover how to love yourself.

ALLOW THE CLIENT
TO INTERPRET

Receiving intuitive impressions while doing Reiki hands-on or distant-healing treatment is often like dreaming someone else's dream. The images flow and change and change again, presenting many symbols, some of them filled with what seems obvious meaning. For the inexperienced Reiki practitioner, the temptation may be great to immediately interpret these symbols and present this analysis to the client as a fait accompli.

How does a client, offered such an analysis, respond?

"I'm sorry, but that just doesn't feel right to me."

"Could you run that by me again? That doesn't quite make sense. . . ."

"*What* did you see? Could you please describe that impression again?"

And when the image is presented to the client, this time without any overlay of interpretation, the client looks perplexed for a moment, then mutters, "That's not what that image means to me. . . ."

If experience is the best teacher, a Reiki practitioner who attempts to interpret intuitive impressions that arise during a hands-on session very quickly learns that this task is best left to the client. Interpretation is work—and it is the client's right to do the emotional and mental work of reflection, understanding, and release in order to claim the most complete and permanent healing.

Why? Consider dream analysis. A dream analyst will tell you that the one who can make the most accurate interpretation of any dream is the dreamer. This is, in part, because the dreamer is the writer, artist, producer, and actor of all parts in every scene of a dream, but there are other reasons as well. Some dreams help the dreamer to process the experiences of each day, absorbing and storing some events into memory, some into the subconscious mind, and discarding others. Some dreams present to conscious awareness those memories that have been stored in the subconscious mind for a time because they were too painful to recall; when the dreamer is ready to face them and heal them, those memories emerge in the symbolic language of dreams. On waking, the dreamer has the choice of deliberately recalling the dream and doing whatever work of healing it seems to demand, or allowing the dream to fade away. The person who chooses to do the dreamwork may reflect on a dream and claim healing, understanding, forgiveness and release, creativity, and greater peace of mind.

These rewards also rightfully belong to the Reiki client willing to do the work of interpreting any intuitive impressions that arise during treatment. While intuitive impressions occasionally arise in the mind of the client receiving Reiki, usually the client is so relaxed that the flow of the energy carries impressions into the more alert mind of the practitioner, to be presented to the client after the treatment. The practitioner's role is somewhat like that of a doctor hearing a patient's confidences; the practitioner is entrusted with the responsibility of listening closely to those thoughts, feelings, images that are communicated by the client, without passing judgment. Yet the responsibility does not end there: the practitioner may then describe whatever impressions have come, without comment, when the client is ready to hear them. Serving in this way, connected through Reiki hands and consciousness to consciousness, is a privilege and a sacred trust. Recognizing this may dissolve the impulse to do the work of interpretation for the client, who comes to the practitioner seeking healing on all levels.

A TOY BOX IN THE MIND

Fortunately, Reiki usually teaches us this lesson with lots of laughter along the way. One August day I taught Reiki I to a student who was completely preoccupied with babies: she and her husband, while hoping to someday conceive their own child, had filed for adoption, and the day after our class they would be bringing home twin boys; she had also recently learned that she was pregnant.

Because I taught her one on one, I had the privilege of being her first client. As she worked at my head, with her hands lightly placed over my forehead, eyes, upper sinuses, and teeth, an image flashed into her mind, which she described to me. She saw a baby's toy, she said: a cone that sits on top of a rocking platform, with several colored doughnuts of progressively smaller sizes. My student told me that in her mind's eye she could see me sitting on the floor with this toy in front of me, and I had all the doughnuts on the cone but one.

"Which one is missing?" I asked.

"The red one."

Strangely enough, I immediately understood what this image was about. I associate the color red with the root chakra, the energy center located at the base of the spine, as described in Indian philosophy. I think of the root chakra as having to do with practical connections to this world.

Under my student's fingertips, the Reiki energy was flowing into a problem area for me: a bone infection above one of my front teeth. I had done a lot of journaling to understand the original cause of the infection, which went all the way back to my childhood. I was ready for the area to be completely healed, but I was missing the one practical element I needed: an endodontist whom I trusted to do the necessary surgery. The impression she described confirmed for me that it was now time for me to find a qualified dental surgeon.

Shortly after this treatment, a friend at a Reikishare mentioned that she had learned of an endodontist, trained in Reiki, who had an office nearby. I called his office the next day and set up an appointment for the surgery. With Reiki friends sending Reiki to me during the operation, it went smoothly; the area of infection was completely removed, and my mouth healed quickly and well.

This experience allowed me to make the point to my Reiki I student that it is important to present any impressions received to the client for interpretation, rather than trying to interpret them yourself. Did the image of the child's toy mean anything to my student? Yes, absolutely! With three babies on the way and a nursery ready, well stocked with toys, she had many associations with this toy. However, the image did not hold the same meaning for her that it did for me—and in this instance I was the client; it was my healing needs that were being served by our session. By describing the image to me and allowing me to make sense of it in terms of my own life, my student enabled me to claim complete healing.

The incident made me think more about how Reiki and intuition work together for healing. In the communion of minds that so often accompanies Reiki healing, one consciousness joins another for a "timeless" moment in time. The images and impressions that float to the surface of the practitioner's awareness are often appealingly simple and innocent. Perhaps this is also due to the nature of the subconscious mind, which psychologists often describe as childlike.

What happened that afternoon, when my Reiki I student received an intuitive impression that had one set of associations for her but another quite different set for me, is typical. Over the years, as I have treated Reiki clients, I have often seen visual images that seemed to have an obvious meaning, but I have stopped trying to second-guess their meaning for my clients. For example, when the image of a pitcher of water and a glass come up, I will still describe it to my client in detail: "I see a tall glass pitcher of sparkling, clear water and an empty glass beside it. It looks refreshing." However, I will not ask, "Do you think you are getting enough water?" Too often, clients for whom this common image has come up have answered, "Oh yes, I drink at least eight glasses a day. Sometimes I feel like I'm going to float away." I no longer presume that the glass is empty because my client needs to drink more water. Now I simply describe what I see and ask, "Does this mean something to you?" or "What do you make of that?"

AN IMPRESSION SUPERIMPOSED ON REALITY

Sometimes the purpose interpretation serves is to guide the client to make a future healing choice, as this story illustrates: At a well-attended Reikishare, with eight practitioners gathered around the table, I found myself seated at the client's head. As I held my hands in first position, a ghostly image began to take form in front of me. Even with my eyes open, I could see Alfred E. Neuman, the freckle-faced, leering cover boy of *MAD Magazine*. Then another form appeared to the right: a covered bridge, which bent in half and drifted over onto Alfred E. Neuman's face, hiding his grin. I had no idea what to make of these impressions, yet they lingered. They continued to float over the client until at last, I asked him, "Does the cover of *MAD Magazine* mean anything to you?"

Without a moment's hesitation, he said, "No."

Still, Alfred E. Neuman and the covered bridge hung shimmering in the air before my eyes.

After about another ten minutes, everyone felt the energy become quiet, and the client got up from the table. He thanked everyone, then looked at me. "I've been thinking about your question," he said. "When I was seventeen or eighteen, I used to draw Alfred E. Neuman in school notebooks all the time."

"Oh, I'm so glad it means something to you," I said, feeling relieved. "Let me tell you about the rest of the impression: I saw a covered bridge—"

Before I could finish my sentence, he interrupted me: "That's easy. I went to the dentist this afternoon, and we talked about whether or not I needed bridge-work done."

I was astounded. This possibility hadn't even occurred to me. It was another wonderful lesson in the importance of allowing the client to interpret any intuitive impressions received while doing Reiki.

Sometimes, of course, the client can't make immediate sense of all the intuitive impressions a practitioner receives and describes during a treatment session. Often, however, by the end of a session, the client will have quietly explored memory and the meaning will have become clear. Occasionally, days later, the practitioner will receive a call from a client, who wants to share the feeling of success that follows when the last puzzle piece falls into place—and the emotional and mental healing issues that arose during the Reiki session are able to be consciously addressed by the client and resolved.

LET THE CLIENT DECIDE

It is indeed a privilege to be a Reiki practitioner and energy worker, bringing healing to the client not only physically, but emotionally, mentally, and spiritually too. Clients who are aware of the potential for healing that Reiki holds can tempt a practitioner to say more about intuitive impressions than seems comfortable or wise.

Mani, a lovely young Indian woman, enjoyed receiving Reiki at the Reikishare. When Kittu, her sixteen-year-old gray tiger cat was diagnosed with a cancerous tumor, she begged me to do Reiki distant healing. As a Reiki practitioner who is neither a doctor nor a nurse practitioner (nor a vet, in this case), I did not want to be put in the position of seeming to diagnose or prescribe. I thought about Mani's request for a few days, and then finally told her that I would send Reiki to her cat and ask to receive impressions of his thoughts and feelings regarding his treatment options: surgery, radiation, or both. I cautioned Mani that whatever impressions I received could, at best, only show future possibilities. I could make no promises, no guarantees, nor I could I "predict" a successful outcome based on any impressions I received. She said that she understood, but would like me to go ahead with the session anyway.

When I connected to her cat through Reiki distant healing, impressions came very quickly, and they were quite clear. I saw her cat receiving radiation treatments and recovering rapidly. He seemed to be impatient to get on with the treatments so that he could then get on with his life. He wanted to have one of Mani's scarves in his cage and a tape of the family chanting their daily prayers for his stay at the veterinary hospital. I saw Mani's cat stretched out comfortably on the scarf, taking comfort from its familiar smell, and enjoying the healing sound vibrations of the chanting.

Mani thanked me for sending Reiki to her cat and for the impressions I relayed. She followed through completely in accord with her cat's wishes as they were suggested by the impressions. He survived the radiation treatments, and recovered quickly and well. "After the treatment," Mani says, "he was like a kitten—so happy, so playful. He was able to do all the things he loved to do before he got sick—have fun outside, hunt mice, play with toys." He enjoyed the life of a happy, healthy cat until his death a year and a half later.

SUGGESTIONS FOR PRACTITIONERS

As you do hands-on or distant healing, be aware that your connection to your client through the Reiki energy occurs in sacred time and space. In that realm, not only does Spirit-guided healing energy flow from your hands into your client's physical body, but also into your client's emotional, mental, and spiritual "bodies," sometimes collectively called the aura or human energy field. With your consciousness joined to your client's in the flow of Reiki energy, impressions may come to you regarding the client's healing needs on any and all of these levels. Your task is simply to describe whatever impressions you do receive and to allow the client the satisfaction of doing the work of interpretation—remembrance, reflection, feeling, and release. This will enable your client to claim more complete healing.

Treat whatever occurs and whatever is discussed during your client sessions as confidential. Properly record impressions received, as well as sensations of the energy, in your client progress notes or journal—and keep your notes or journal in a safe place. Value the privilege of being a holistic treatment provider.

Finally, enjoy the awareness of unity that is revealed through the experience of Reiki. Whether or not any intuitive impressions arise as you treat your client, the meditative quality of that experience is the dream of sages and saints.

NOW YOU

In order to parallel the experience of a client who is offered an interpretation by a Reiki practitioner, share one of your dreams with a friend. Ask for an interpretation. Listen attentively to your friend's response. How similar is your friend's interpretation to your own? Does the friend's interpretation offer any new insights? Does it make you doubt your own interpretation? Has the experience of considering your friend's interpretation of your dream made you feel empowered or disempowered? If you feel more satisfied with your own interpretation, remind yourself that the dreamer is the best dream analyst of his or her own dream.

Resolve not to impose your interpretation on intuitive impressions that arise as you treat your clients. Allow your client the richly rewarding task of making sense of these messages. Let the client claim complete healing.

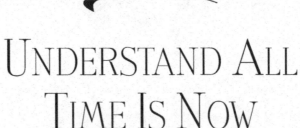

10

UNDERSTAND ALL
TIME IS NOW

Past, present, and future are all one in the realm of sacred time and space in which Reiki healing is offered and received. As the practitioner's awareness becomes focused on the flow of the Reiki energy, the practitioner begins to feel better: more relaxed, centered, and peaceful. In fact, much more occurs: with attention focused on following the infinitely healing energy of Reiki, perception expands toward the infinite in support of healing. Suddenly, or gradually, the practitioner becomes aware that certain barriers that are taken for granted during ordinary awareness seem to be gone: for example, Reiki-charged hands may seem to melt into the client, as if the boundary between self and other has dissolved.

Similarly, there may be a mental and emotional contact that is so gentle, so deeply healing, that the fact that it radically transcends ordinary awareness causes no concern. Through this Reiki-charged connection, information from the client's past, present, or future may enter the practitioner's awareness in the form of intuitive impressions, if the sharing of that information in some way supports healing. Although it is sometimes apparent to the practitioner that the information, "encrypted" in the dreamlike form of intuitive impressions, relates to a particular time, usually the client must figure this out.

LESSONS ABOUT TIME: SEEING THE PAST

While the experience described in chapter 7, in which I received intuitive impressions of a friend's car accident six months before as I sent him Reiki distant healing, had a profound impact on my understanding of Reiki's ability to heal across time, there were many more lessons to come. During the 1990s, experiences during Reiki treatments on my regular client, friend, and graduate school mentor, Professor Daniel O'Hara, helped me to understand this principle of practice.

When Dan first began coming for Reiki treatments he was suffering from work-related stress, high blood pressure, and old, incompletely healed back injuries that were the result of being in a serious car accident several years before. He came for treatments every other week, for two-hour sessions, over a period of three years. Initially he welcomed the sense of relaxation that Reiki gave him; he was happy to discover that the catnap he routinely caught on the bodywork table was just his body's first response to Reiki. During the days that followed a treatment, he would feel calmer and more alert, in a better mood, and his blood pressure would be down. After a few months of treatment he began to notice that the old injuries from the accident were bothering him much less.

During one of these sessions, as I treated him in silence with my hands on his lower back, a rather startling image flashed into my mind: a sunny-side egg frying on a sidewalk. Since the feeling through my hands on Dan's back could have been described at that moment as "sizzling hot," this image made sense to me as an indication of the intensity of the Reiki energy radiating into him, and it subtly reminded me to keep my hands in place until it had done its work of healing. Neither of us was concerned by this intensity; we both knew from experience that the heat we felt would not physically harm him in any way and it indicated the degree of his need for healing. This single afternoon's treatment with the Reiki brought these damaged muscle fibers back into balance.

Dan continued to come for regular treatments and, much to our shared surprise, the Reiki energy brought up even older injuries for healing. One afternoon, as I again worked on his lower back and hip, my quiet meditation on the light of Reiki was abruptly ended by a sudden image of a uniformed baseball player sliding into third base. Startled out of my reverie, I asked, "Have you watched any baseball on television in the last day or two?"

"No," he said.

I described what I had seen and asked another question: "Did you ever play baseball?"

"No," he said again.

We settled back into the comforting silence of the treatment process. Over the next twenty minutes I moved my hands through the few remaining positions and closed the session. Dan relaxed on the table for another couple of minutes and then rolled onto his side and sat up.

"I've been thinking about what you saw," he said. "I played baseball as a child, up until I was in the third grade. I guess I was about nine years old. We had a game at school and I slid into a base on that hip. I bruised it pretty badly. After that I didn't play any more. I sat on the sidelines."

"So the image did mean something to you. . . ."

"Yes. I just had to think back far enough in time to remember."

"Well I imagine you'll feel quite a bit better after this," I assured him. He did—and that was the day he decided that he wanted to learn Reiki himself.

When information like this comes into my awareness during a Reiki session, I look upon it as a validation of the healing process and a reminder to the client to reflect on the past to discover what may still need to be released. Did Dan suffer more than physical injury to his hip some forty years earlier? He told me after this session that his injury during the baseball game was significant in another way: after it occurred he decided to avoid after-school sports and concentrate on his studies. So this incident marked a turning point in his life; he fell into being "bookish" on his way to becoming a university professor and scholar. The Reiki healed the old injury and, in reminding him of the injury's impact on his life, validated his choice.

Whether intuitive impressions come during a hands-on treatment or a distant-healing session, it is always best to let the client consider them and decide if they are linked to the present, the past, the future. Unlike a digital camera or a video image, intuitive Reiki impressions do not bear a date and time indicator at the bottom of the picture. They can be accurate and meaningful but still not identifiable to the practitioner. Allow the client to make sense of them. When we connect to our clients through Reiki, we meet them in the realm of Spirit, all-knowing and all-present. A decade ago, yesterday, tomorrow—all are one; all chronological time, as we think of it, is now.

LESSONS ABOUT TIME: SEEING TOMORROW

As I teach Reiki, I sometimes have the opportunity to see students gain this same realization about time through their experiences. In July 2000, Reiki Master Carole Koch read my book *Traditional Reiki for Our Times*. She was intrigued by the distant-healing method I described learning from Reverend Beth Gray, which emphasized intuition in Reiki practice. Carole decided that she wanted very much to add this particular healing technique to her Reiki practice. She called me and arranged to become recertified in Reiki II, the distant-healing course, in a private class.

Toward the end of the class I offered Carole the opportunity to practice on a client unknown to her. I gave her a photograph of my mother and father taken as a formal portrait for their fiftieth wedding anniversary. I told Carole my mother's name and asked her to send distant healing, jotting down in a notebook any impressions she received during the session, which lasted about forty-five minutes.

At the completion of the treatment, we exchanged feedback on our distant-healing clients. Carole told me she had few impressions: that the woman she had treated was wasting away, that she should drink a lot of nutritious milk shakes, and that there was a dark red tube in her chest wall that led into her heart. I explained to her that she had been sending Reiki to my mother, who was seriously ill, and thanked her. Then I described my mother's condition: she had recently been admitted to the hospital and was being fed intravenously because she had lost a lot of weight, for reasons as yet unknown; before going into the hospital my mother had tried to drink milk shakes for their protein and mineral contents and high calories. I could not tell Carole what the dark red tube was; I had no idea what it meant.

When I got home that night after the class I learned that, during the afternoon, as Carole had been sending Reiki to my mother, her doctors had been in consultation with a cardiologist. The next day a cardiac surgeon (who happened to be a Reiki practitioner herself) would do surgery to insert a pacemaker.

Once the operation was completed and my mother was in recovery, I called Carole to let her know the reason for her impression of the "dark red tube." Though she had only a few impressions, all were accurate, and she had accessed not only information about my mother's past medical history and present condition, but also her immediate future. This event confirmed again the all-knowing, all-now quality of Spirit, source for Reiki's healing power and source for intuitive guidance.

RIDING WAVES OF REIKI INTO THE FUTURE

Massage therapist Lynn Deemer discovered Reiki during the course of her training at the Pennsylvania School of Massage Therapy. She loved the idea of being able to provide clients with deep healing while her own hands and arms were quiet, simply flowing with Reiki energy.

About a year after taking the basic course Lynn decided to learn distant healing. Like many of my classes, hers was small: only one other student, a Bucks County artist, was registered for the class. For one of the practice exercises I required these two practitioners to send distant healing to each other and to share any intuitive impressions they received. While most of the impressions the artist received and described made sense to Lynn, one completely puzzled her: an image of a cowboy on a bucking bronco, holding on to his hat. Lynn had no idea what this image meant.

On the day following the class, an old friend of Lynn's invited her to go down to Atlantic City the next day on a casino bus. Since Lynn had no massage clients scheduled for the day she accepted the invitation.

Early the next morning the two boarded a local tour bus for the two-and-a-half hour ride. They happily passed the time in conversation, catching up on each other's lives. When they disembarked from the bus in the parking lot of the Wild West Casino and entered the lobby, Lynn immediately spotted a fifteen-foot-high statue of a rodeo cowboy on a rearing horse, his hat held high. Lynn realized she faced the reality of the intuitive impression her fellow Reiki II student had shared the day before: here was the future become the present moment, full of possibility.

"This is it!" she told her friend. "This is where I want to play."

Fortunately, her friend was glad to spend the day in a single casino. Lynn won $400 playing at a slot machine, more money than she had ever won in her life.

"This is so cool!" she told me afterward, thrilled to have been given Reiki's gentle guidance to lay claim to a bit of abundance along her spiritual path.

Again, Reiki had accessed information along the continuum of chronological time as if all time is now, as indeed it is to Spirit. The opportunity to play in a casino and win, signaled by the image of the rodeo cowboy riding high, was just that—an opportunity, not a destiny. Lynn simply recognized it as such and chose, by free will, to take advantage of it.

SUGGESTIONS FOR PRACTITIONERS

Whether you are doing hands-on Reiki or distant healing, understand that any intuitive impressions you receive via the flow of Reiki energy may relate to the past, the present, or the possible future. If you are uncertain, and it is possible to ask the client for comment, please do. If it is not possible or appropriate to ask the client for clarification, then ask the Reiki energy to show the same information in another way—or ask Spirit for clarification. If the answer that comes intuitively is that the impression shows you an event that has already occurred, ask another question: How recently did this event occur? An answer may or may not be forthcoming. Accept whatever does come with gratitude.

Do remember to relax. Remind yourself of the Reiki principles (in particular,

"Just for today, do not worry") before you begin a treatment. This will bring you into accord with the practice of traditional Japanese Reiki practitioners in the Usui Reiki Ryoho Gakkai, who recite the Reiki principles in silence as a brief meditation before beginning a Reiki treatment.

Finally, know that the Reiki energy, through every treatment, continues to teach you—as it continues to teach all practitioners long after the official close of their Reiki class.

NOW YOU

Consider the Dalai Lama, who instructs his followers, lifetime after lifetime, where to look for him in his next incarnation. What could be more comforting to the Tibetan Buddhist monks who devote themselves to prayer, meditation, and service than the knowledge that the titular and spiritual head of their order, soon after his death, will be born again, replete with all his wisdom, in a certain place, at a certain time? They wait years, and then they seek the child, test him, and discover once again His Holiness.

Before your next client session, ask your client if he or she is interested in being made aware of any intuitive impressions you receive. If your client says yes, then ask if he or she would prefer to be told of impressions as they arise during the session or at the end of the session. Honor this request. Set your intention to be open to impressions from the past, present, and future. Then relax and enjoy the experience.

When you describe your impressions, let the client know that they may be associated with the past, the present, or the future, so it is perfectly fine if an impression doesn't make immediate sense. It may have to do with an event that occurred so long ago that the client has forgotten about it, or it may have to do with an event which has not yet occurred—and that may never occur, depending on the client's use of free will.

When you conclude your session with your client, take a few moments to record your client progress notes and any impressions you intuitively received.

Note the impressions that the client recognized as belonging in the past or the present, as well as those that were unknown.

Once you make a habit of setting your intention to be open to receive intuitive impressions from the past, present, and future during a Reiki session, you will find they occur more frequently. Recording them in the client's progress notes or a journal is a way to indicate that you value these impressions. This appreciation is also likely to increase the quantity and quality of intuitive impressions you receive as you do Reiki.

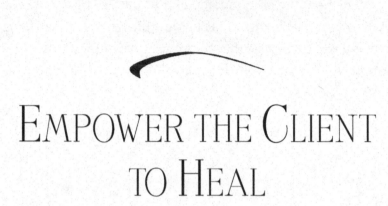

11

EMPOWER THE CLIENT
TO HEAL

The realization that you are becoming more intuitive as a Reiki practitioner—and better able to help your clients to claim complete healing—is a comfort to the soul and a joy to the heart. Yet as you become more capable of offering your clients impressions they can use to gain valuable self-understanding and healing insights, there is a danger: some clients may begin to look to you for answers that are best learned through their own efforts. If you allow this dependence to develop and to continue, you take a risk as well: you may become proud of "your" power, and in that arrogance you may lose ground on your spiritual path. The harmony you have sought, the peace of mind, the compassion, may slip away, as you confront and evade your own ego and its attachments.

Let go. Breathe and relax into the flow of the Reiki energy and do all that you can to empower your client to claim complete, permanent healing. In the past, when you have had a Reiki client who asked more of you as a practitioner than you felt qualified, willing, ready, and able to give, you may have set boundaries and offered resources. For example, you may have encouraged clients who wanted to overstay their session time to leave with a gentle knock on the door and an announcement: "Millie, I'm sorry, but time's up. I'd love to let you relax on the table for the rest of the afternoon, but my next client is due in ten minutes." Or you may have said to a client who cried with relief during a session, and afterward began to tell you about the difficulties of his personal life, "I'm glad that you experienced some emotional healing today, but I'm not qualified as a counselor or therapist. Would you like me to recommend someone who could offer you that support?"

When you practice intuitive Reiki, you need to be able to set boundaries as well, so that you empower the client to claim healing and, at the same time, discourage the client from depending on you for guidance. A client who is emotionally distraught, unable to think clearly and calmly or to make a decision with confidence, may feel Reiki's healing and want to put you in charge of solving all life's problems. Don't be tempted. Refuse. To do otherwise is to reinforce the role of the victim, who does not feel responsible for scenarios at play in his or her life, and that someone may be abusive and manipulative. Clearly, reinforcing such a pattern is not in the client's best interests and is directly opposed to the purposes of Reiki: to bring healing, empowerment, enlightenment.

Instead, you might remind the client of inner resources: self-knowledge, character strengths, inborn talents, acquired skills, remembered accomplishments—and of free will. Help the client recognize the healing value of creative self-expression: journaling, drawing, painting, dancing, making music, throwing clay, sculpting, cooking, baking, sewing. If it seems appropriate, point out the detoxifying, cleansing effects of physical exercise: a daily walk or swim, a hard run, a forceful sweeping of the kitchen. For clients who are open to spirituality and religion, acknowledge that prayer and meditation, the practice of forgiveness, and the practice of gratitude can be life changing. Be willing to recommend books that might be instructive or offer insight. Finally, be able to suggest support groups, pastoral counselors, therapists, and other professionals who will be glad to listen to the client's concerns, enabling the client to continue the healing work initiated in intuitive Reiki sessions to the point of closure.

As for your own spiritual healing as you become more proficient with intuitive Reiki, remember that, as poet T. S. Eliot said, "The wisdom of humility is endless." It is the Reiki energy that heals your client; it is the Reiki energy that presents to your awareness information for your client in the form of intuitive impressions. Like images from dreams, which half reveal and half conceal their meaning, these impressions can best be interpreted and understood by the client. By simply describing these impressions, when appropriate, with accuracy and without judgment, you invite your client to engage more actively in the emotional and mental work of healing. This empowers the client.

HELPING A REIKI FRIEND
CLAIM COMPLETE HEALING

My friend Terry is as dear to me as a sister. We met in 1980, when I attended a science fiction convention for the first time. In a large, mostly empty auditorium she sat alone, dressed in a business suit, her head bent over her needlepoint as she waited for a panel discussion to begin. Fleeing from the strangers dressed in Klingon warrior and wood-elf costumes, I found a seat beside her and introduced myself. Within five minutes we had discovered that we shared the same alma mater, an interest in archaeology and art history—and we were laughing.

After I learned Reiki in 1987, Terry was one of the first people I told about the class. When I offered to give her a Reiki treatment she accepted. On the basis of that experience and my enthusiasm, she decided to learn Reiki herself the next time Reiki Master Beth Gray came to our area. Since then we have "been there" for one another through hardships and happy occasions—and our friendship has grown even stronger.

One evening Terry called me in tears. She had just returned from her annual visit to her gynecologist. The gynecologist had palpated a small mass in her left breast; a mammogram performed the same day had shown a pleomorphic calcium mass in the right breast. The gynecologist had scheduled further tests: doctors would do a guided aspiration under ultrasound on the left breast in three weeks and an extensive computerized imaging test on the other in six weeks. Nothing could be done sooner because the suburban Philadelphia hospital where the tests were scheduled was working with a reduced staff, due to summer vacations.

I listened in shocked silence. Then, when she paused to hear what I would say, I said a quick prayer for guidance. "Terry, that's good news!" I told her.

"What do you mean it's good news?" she protested.

"That delay in the testing means we have more time to do Reiki. Let's make a treatment plan."

"You're right," Terry said. I heard her take a deep, slow breath and a long, relaxing exhale.

"If I leave here right now and get on the road, I should be able to get to your house in about an hour," I told her.

"Okay," she said, her voice calmer now. "I'll see you soon."

I set down the receiver, collected purse and keys, and then paused, listening to the voice of my intuition: bring crayons and newsprint. Okay. I rooted around and discovered the crayons in a drawer and brought the roll of newsprint out of the closet. Then, juggling these items, I went out the door. I got in my car and drove to Philadelphia, pushing through traffic with my speedometer needle hovering just on the other side of the legal limit. While I drove I prayed and thought, asking for guidance about how to help Terry get through this crisis. When I arrived I hugged my friend and asked if she would like me to do Reiki on her as we talked. She nodded.

Because she did not have a bodywork table, and I had not brought mine along, she stretched out on her bed, face up. I sat on a chair beside the bed and extended my arms to treat her, both hands-on and hands off—in the energy field. We talked—and continued the treatment—for hours.

For both of us, now with years of experience as Reiki practitioners, the treatment option of first choice was Reiki itself. Terry and her husband, both Reiki practitioners, could do hands-on Reiki daily; close friends Michael, Leslie, and I could send Reiki in absentia each day to support Terry's healing process now and forward in time to the day of the hospital tests. On the day of each test, Leslie and I could accompany Terry to the hospital, send Reiki to her as she underwent the procedures, and be there afterward to provide whatever emotional support she needed. It was a good plan, and Terry visibly relaxed as she understood the amount of help she could ask for and receive.

With a plan for regular hands-on and distant-healing treatments in place, we asked ourselves what other changes Terry could make that might be helpful. We were both aware that caffeine can contribute to fibrous breast tissue. Without feeling any sense of sacrifice, Terry could eliminate tea and chocolate. She could drink more water and increase her intake of vitamin C and cruciferous vegetables. These were all simple, practical changes she could make in her lifestyle that might help.

Because we were both students trained in Reiki I and II by Beth Gray, we also remembered the emphasis that Beth placed on applying Reiki to the original cause of an injury, illness, or condition to encourage complete, permanent healing. We understood that this "original cause" might be an event that triggered emotions that were quickly repressed. As Beth's gift to us, along with our certificates of completion we had both received a wonderful punch-out human anatomy book and a little blue book that contained Louise Hay's affirmations for healing, *Heal Your Body: The Mental Causes for Physical Illness and the Metaphysical Way to Overcome Them*. We knew that the physical breast was often associated with issues of mothering, nurturing, caring.

"Can you think of any events that might have occurred within the last year or so that were about nurturing for you?" I asked Terry.

"Absolutely," she said. "Taking care of my cats this year as they were dying was about nurturing. And I know I haven't really grieved for them."

I thought of the three beautiful cats Terry had loved and cared for into their old ages, who had died within months of one another from unrelated causes. The kitten she had adopted at the SPCA, hoping it would heal the ache in her heart, had turned out to have an undiagnosed infection that took his life within a few weeks. I felt her sadness and sat in silence as she delved into the grief she'd been holding at bay.

Eventually I asked if the timing of this event might be significant to her in any other way. I knew from past conversations that she hadn't gotten along well with her mother, and that her mother had died as a relatively young woman. Could she be the same age as her mother had been when she had died?

She shook her head. No, she told me, she wasn't the same age, although she was close to it, and she certainly did have unresolved issues with her mother.

"Do you want to talk about them?" I asked.

"I want to think about them," she said. I accepted this in silence.

"We both know that you need to find a way to express these feelings," I finally said.

"Yes," she said, sniffling. "I don't want to stuff them down any more. I don't want to have 'issues in my tissues.' I want to get the grief out. I want to get it off my chest." She gestured toward her breasts and away, in a sweeping motion, then realized what she had done and laughed.

"I'm here, Terry, and I'll listen, if you want to talk."

She was comforted by this. She told me the story of each of the four cats, their illnesses, the difficulties of their deaths, the sadness she had felt with each one's passing. Sometimes she cried, then reached for a tissue to wipe away her tears so that she could continue. I listened.

When she finished her account she seemed relieved and more in control.

"Feel better?" I asked.

She nodded.

"Do you think that's all the grief you have bottled up?"

She shook her head. "There's more. I can feel it. It was good to talk—I feel better now, lighter, calmer, but I haven't completed the grieving yet."

"I had an idea, just before I left my house, about how you might be able to express and release some of those feelings," I told her.

She looked at me with curiosity. "What's the idea?"

"Well, I know that you enjoy painting in oil, and I also know that you are a perfectionist, and that most of your oil paintings take a long time to complete—a year or so . . ."

She smiled, "Or two or three . . ."

"So how about using your artistic talent to express some of those feelings you have bottled up inside, but without being a perfectionist?"

"How could I do that?" she asked, baffled.

"You know those drawings that kids do on newsprint with crayon that end up on people's refrigerators? I thought that you might try using crayons on newsprint and giving yourself just ten minutes to complete a drawing—like one of those quick, timed drawings in an art class—so it isn't about making the drawing perfect or just right . . ." I trailed off, uncertain how she would take this suggestion.

"I could do that!" she said. "I think I would even like doing that—just dashing off a drawing each day about my cats, or about my mother, or about dying. Do you think I could call you and tell you about what I draw?"

I smiled. "I would be happy to hear about your drawings. Talking about them might be another way to help you to release those feelings, too."

She nodded. "And I could put the drawings on the refrigerator and that would remind me to think about what happened with my cats and with my mother and how it made me feel. As I understood, I could let those feelings go, too." She looked at me and sighed. "But there's a problem."

"What's that?"

"I don't have crayons and newsprint."

"Yes, you do," I said. "I had some crayons in a drawer and a roll of newsprint in my closet. Now they're yours."

She laughed, delighted. "Thank you."

"I'll be expecting to hear about your drawings."

"You will, don't worry!"

During the weeks before the aspiration Terry drew every day and posted her drawings on the refrigerator to reflect on. She called me often to tell me about the drawings and what she had learned from them. Unlike the subjects of her oil paintings, which she researched and attempted to represent in a realistic way, the subjects of her drawings were her feelings—shadowy, violent, sad, angry, happy, confused. When she gave herself permission to draw her feelings she freed herself up to doodle, to draw dreamlike forms, even to add on balloons for speech, comic strip style. The drawings proved to be catalysts for real emotional healing, as any form of creative expression—music, dance, journaling, or other artwork—can be.

Three weeks into the treatment plan Leslie and I accompanied Terry to the hospital. We sent Reiki to Terry from the waiting room as she underwent the guided aspiration on her left breast. Our hands were intensely active—by the time the procedure was completed we both realized that it had probably been quite painful. When Terry emerged from the testing area, still in her gown, she looked tear-streaked but satisfied. "The lump turned out to be a fluid-filled cyst," she told us, "which the surgeon has sent down to the lab." She sighed. "It was a painful procedure—the doctors had to keep switching needles and probing at different angles to try to reach it. Even the doctors were surprised at what I tolerated. I think the only reason that I managed to get through it was the Reiki. Thank you both."

"We're glad to help," Leslie said.

"We'll be back for the next test, too," I assured her.

Later that afternoon, at home, Terry received a phone call from the lab: everything had tested negative.

During the next three weeks Terry continued to treat herself with Reiki, use affirmations, watch her diet, and do her crayon drawings. Her husband treated her with Reiki hands-on, and Michael, Leslie, and I continued to send Reiki distant healing.

On the day the computerized imaging test on Terry's right breast was scheduled to take place, Leslie and I again accompanied Terry to the hospital to provide on-site Reiki support. Since this test involved no incisions and no needle punctures, Terry faced it in better spirits.

Two hours after she entered the testing area she reappeared with a big smile on her face. "The doctors are all inside poring over the images and scratching their heads. They can't find anything wrong!" she told us, her smile turning into a grin. "All they see is normal distribution of calcium throughout the breast."

This experience taught everyone involved many lessons: about the healing power of our joined hands; the opportunity for profound healing to occur between the time a test or medical procedure is scheduled and the time it is actually performed; the value of listening to Reiki-guided intuition; the importance of empowering the client to claim complete, permanent healing on all levels.

SUPPORTING A CLIENT'S DECISION

The same summer that Terry called on me for Reiki help, a nurse whom I knew through the local chapter of the American Holistic Nurses Association asked me if I would be willing to treat her as a client. Of course, I agreed. Before her first session I asked if she had any particular concerns. Yes, she told me. She had a small, palpable mass in her right breast, and her doctor had advised a biopsy right away. She had put him off. She had told her doctor that she wanted to have an opportunity to treat herself with complementary medicine before undergoing the surgeon's knife. He had frowned at her and warned her that she was taking a serious risk with her health. She had bargained with him: if she was able to shrink the mass using Reiki, therapeutic touch, and other holistic healing methods, would he reconsider the biopsy? Shaking his head, he had told her to return in two months, and then he would reexamine her and make his recommendation.

Over that two-month period the nurse treated herself daily using Reiki, therapeutic touch, forgiveness meditations, affirmations. I also treated her several times with Reiki. Finally, at one of our last sessions, she asked, "Please, tell me what your impressions about this. Is the mass smaller? I think it is. Even the doctor thinks it feels smaller, but he still wants me to have the biopsy. I don't want to have it. I think I can heal this myself."

I scratched my head, uncomfortable with being asked to make this kind of evaluation. It felt too much like being asked to diagnose and prescribe, guided by intuition. Finally, I said, "Look, I'll tell you what I feel, but I won't tell you what I think you should do. You have to decide that, guided by your own common sense and your own intuition."

"That's fair," she said.

"I agree with you that the mass feels smaller and seems to be drawing less energy."

"That's what I think, too."

"But if I were in your place, and my doctor was telling me to have a biopsy, I would have the biopsy. That's what I would do. But I'm not in your place, and I can't make that decision for you. You're a nurse and a holistic healer. You've seen the procedure in the operating room. You know more about what a biopsy entails and what it accomplishes than I ever have or will. You are going to have to decide whether or not to have the procedure for yourself."

She looked at me and nodded, her mind already made up. "I'm not going to have it. I'm going to keep working with complementary medicine to get this under control."

"You're a braver woman than I am."

"I just feel really confident that I can heal this with the skills and resources I have."

150

Now I know that she was right. At the time, the most empowering gesture that I could make was to remind her that no one else could make such a difficult decision for her; she had to make it alone. Perhaps her willingness to do so, combined with her determination to do the work of emotional healing that the situation required, helped her become the healthy—and much happier—woman she is today.

ACKNOWLEDGING SELF-DETERMINATION

Several years ago, when I learned that a professor of mine was hospitalized for the second time within five years for a recurrence of colon cancer, I sent Reiki distant healing. Through the intuitive Reiki connection I asked him how I could best help him to recover. I saw him sitting up in his hospital bed, wearing a loose-fitting hospital gown, smiling. He said, "Send me Reiki for a few minutes every day for the next seven days. That's it. That will be enough."

I was shocked. He had asked so little, and yet he had been so precise in his request. So for the next seven days I sent him Reiki distant healing. Sometimes I did this just before I myself fell asleep, struggling to keep my eyes open until the energy shifted in my hands and I was sure he had received enough for deep, accelerated healing.

He asked so little during that first distant-healing session—and yet, more than a decade later, he remains cancer-free. Sometimes the way to empower a client to claim complete healing is to listen to our hands, listen to the client's requests, and honor them. Let the client, who is himself also guided by an inner knowing that issues from his soul's connection to Spirit, be self-determining.

SUGGESTIONS FOR PRACTITIONERS

Recall someone who did you the kindness of putting into your hands the tools you needed to accomplish something important on your own. Remember how good you felt as you gradually learned that acquiring this skill or reaching this goal was within your power? You felt confident. You felt capable. You felt more sure of yourself—of your identity and your purpose. Be willing to offer your clients the same kindness by acknowledging the importance of their positive attitude toward their own healing. Reflect back to them the value of their inner resources. Encourage their active participation in the healing process.

NOW YOU

Be prepared to supply clients with tools that can help them to interpret the intuitive impressions that arise during a Reiki session. You might keep a dictionary of dream symbols on hand, as well as a selection of books about other symbols in nature: flowers, trees, animals. (Gretchen Scoble and Ann Field's *The Meaning of Flowers* and Ted Andrews' *Animal-Speak* and *Animal Wise* sit close at hand, on my bookshelf.)

Remind your client that the symbolism of dreams—and of intuitive Reiki impressions—is often very personal. A client who has an aromatherapy practice may understand you receiving the scent of lavender during a session in an entirely different way than one who just painted her six-year-old daughter's bedroom lavender at her daughter's request. Refuse to do the work of interpretation for the client; instead, encourage the client to engage mentally and emotionally with the imagery and other impressions that come up during the Reiki session. Sometimes it requires conscious, willing reflection and remembrance to release repressed anger, fear, and pain, and to realize the importance of forgiveness.

Help your client to understand that the work of healing old emotional, mental, and spiritual hurts often takes time and may require professional support you are not qualified to provide. Describe to clients who are responsive to these suggestions how creative expression and journaling can support the emotional healing process, and encourage them to try out these activities. Get to know the local mental health care providers, pastoral counselors, and support groups in your area, and assemble a list of names, addresses, and phone numbers that you can give to clients who might benefit from one-on-one counseling or another kind of therapeutic support.

12

EXPANDING PRACTICE: ASKING FOR GUIDANCE

When someone asks—or prays to Spirit—for guidance, unless the request has been made with all kinds of restrictions in place, then that guidance can come at any time, in any way. Actor Jim Carrey made a movie called *Bruce Almighty* in which he plays Bruce Nolan, a TV reporter whose life is in disarray. In one scene he is driving down the highway and complaining to God, asking for a sign. Just in front of him is a dump truck with a full load of bright yellow "caution" and "warning" signs. Even though Bruce Nolan looks right at them he doesn't get the message. Of course, his situation continues to get worse.

Most people are not in the habit of looking for signs in the external world. Yet for Reiki practitioners and all holistic healers, this is a wise habit to cultivate. This world is vibrantly alive, and the apparent solidity of matter an illusion, simply the dance of atoms slowed to the point that we perceive form—for a time. The constant in our world is energy, which, physicists tell us, can be influenced by the power of thought. Has humanity created God by a consensus of thought across all of recorded history? Or is there, somehow encoded in the human genome, the instruction within each individual to create the thought of

God? For many people who feel an innate knowing that there is a God or some benevolent, guiding, higher power, the answer to this puzzle does not matter (For those curious about this as a quantum-physics puzzle, see the movie *What the BLΣΣP Do We Know!?*)

Reiki is not a religion. In both the Western tradition and the Japanese, Reiki has been taught, for generations, in a secular way. Yet most Reiki practitioners soon have the evidence of their own eyes and ears and other senses assuring them that yes, something healing has occurred, something that is far beyond a physicians' skill to accomplish and the practitioner's intellect to comprehend. At this point the Reiki practitioner may begin to acknowledge the spirit of Reiki, to admit the possibility that a benevolent, guiding higher power works through Reiki-attuned hands to bring profound healing.

For many practitioners this acknowledgment through personal experience is a spiritual healing—a gentle readjustment of their ideas of God, an antidote to lost faith, an evolution not incompatible with religion but not defined by it either. With this expanded awareness of the presence of Spirit in all that is, it becomes natural to begin to look for other evidence of that presence outside the Reiki treatment room.

Here is a quick example. Three years after I learned Reiki I went through a difficult legal proceeding. On the day that the case finally came to court and the judge ruled in my favor, as I walked down the courthouse steps for the last time I saw a bottle cap. I leaned down to pick it up so that others did not slip on it. It turned out to be an Elliot's Juice bottle cap, with a quotation from the poet Rumi printed inside in very small letters: "Faith is the bird that sings when the dawn is still dark." I pocketed the bottle cap and brushed away tears, knowing that here was a "sign" from the universe: my faith had been rewarded, yet I would need to maintain it through difficulties still ahead. I was filled with gratitude for this token of support.

Some people might think that I was silly to read so much into such a "coincidence." Yet I have learned, over time, to value coincidence, to accept the definition that a so-called coincidence is "a miracle in which God wishes to remain anonymous." When coincidence after coincidence occurs I consider the possibility that I am faced with synchronicity: a concurrence of forces, a juxtaposition of events, people, ideas strongly supporting a particular choice. I pay attention. I ask for guidance, and I am alert that I may receive it in any form. When I do notice something that seems a sign I allow myself to be guided by it, to act upon it.

In the summer of 1998, shortly after *Traditional Reiki for Our Times* was published, I became involved in a relationship with a man, a fellow Reiki practitioner whom I met at a Reikishare. The relationship stalled soon after it was begun, and I became depressed that it was going nowhere. Yet I stayed in the relationship for years, saying nothing about my unhappiness. Eventually the universe confronted me with my fears through three encounters with Mack trucks that took place over about five weeks. In the first experience I felt myself squeezed off the road as a truck veered into my lane. In the second instance my car was physically pushed backward by a Mack truck reversing down a hill, its driver unaware of my tiny hatchback behind him. In the third I slowed to a stop behind a Mack truck pulling to a halt at a stop sign, but it stopped sooner than I expected and I rear-ended the truck. My car was totaled, while the Mack truck did not even have a paint scratch.

These three events, so closely occurring, seemed more than coincidence. What was the universe saying to me that I was ignoring to the extent that the message now had to be delivered by eighteen-wheelers? What did Mack trucks represent to me? In the days that followed the accident, while I waited for the insurance company to okay repairs or declare my car a loss, I had time alone to think. Trucks, big trucks. Race cars. Toys for men. Where in my life was I being stalled or pushed back by the male energy? As soon as I interpreted these events as if they were a dream, I knew the answer: the lack of any future in my relationship was hurting me, scaring me, and holding me back. I gathered my courage to have a conversation that I did not want to have with my partner. We became engaged, but sadly, that phase of our relationship also became stalled, and I broke it off, lesson learned: pay attention to feelings, speak up, say what is in the heart.

As a result of incidents like this I teach my Reiki II students that guidance is available to all of us, at all times, not only as we do Reiki. Pay attention to the whispers and we may be able to avoid wake-up calls. We can ask for guidance by connecting to Mikao Usui, Chujiro Hayashi, and Hawayo Takata through the Reiki distant-healing process, but guidance can also come to us in a dream, in a glimpse of hawk overhead, in a line of melody overheard through an open window. There is no need to strive or to struggle to receive such guidance. It is all around us. When we feel confused or concerned about some issue, all we need to do is ask for help—ask for clarity, wisdom, peace of mind, direction—and pay attention to what happens over the course of the next few hours or days. We will receive the help we ask for.

RECEIVING THE GUIDANCE OF THE TEACHERS

When Reiki Master Beth Gray suddenly retired from teaching, due to a stroke, in the fall of 1992, those of us who had assisted again and again at her classes in Pennsylvania and New Jersey sent her Reiki—and missed her as a beloved teacher. Years passed. In her absence and in the absence of any Reiki Master to whom I might take my questions, I began to think about using the "talking symbol" to connect to the teachers, to Beth, and also to Hawayo Takata, Chujiro Hayashi, and Mikao Usui.

Because I had spiritual healing to do around the issue of unworthiness, it took months before I worked up the courage to try. Eventually, however, I did try—and I discovered that these teachers are willing, even eager, to answer questions about Reiki and to provide guidance on any other issues that they perceive as important to a practitioner's ability to live a happy and healthy life.

One January day I first connected to Hawaya Takata, offering Reiki healing and asking for her guidance. As I sat with my hands raised up to heart level, my palms a few inches apart, picturing her, feeling the flow of Reiki, many impressions flashed through my mind. I heard a voice, which I imagined to be hers, encouraging me to more practice. Finally, she said, "And by the way, your income taxes this year will be around $600, and you will have the money to pay them." I was shocked. I had not asked for guidance about my financial situation through this Reiki connection; I was concerned whether or not connecting with these teachers at all was appropriate. I didn't want to abuse or misuse this connection in any way.

Yet Takata's words comforted me. I had been anxious for weeks about preparing my income taxes. I hadn't started filling out the forms, and I was worried that on my salary as an adjunct college instructor I wouldn't have the money to pay whatever taxes were due. When I prepared my income tax forms in early April of that year and tallied up the amount due, I discovered that I owed $604—and I did have enough money in the bank to pay that amount. To me, this was an amazing—and very personal—validation, and a lesson in what kind of questions may be appropriate to take to the teachers.

(I have since learned that, during her lifetime, Takata thought a sense of financial security necessary to maintain good health. You can listen to her speak about this issue and tell wonderful stories of her experiences with Reiki on the audio tape, "Takata Speaks: Reiki Stories, Volume 1," available for purchase online from the John Harvey Gray Center for Reiki Healing, www.mv.com/ipusers/reiki/. This tape was created and digitally remastered from recordings made by the Grays during Takata's visits to teach classes in their home in the 1970s.)

After this first experience I became more comfortable with the idea of talking to the ancestral teachers. I learned to call them in individually and together. With each experience of connecting to the teachers I came to know them in a much more personal way. The reverence and awe that I had felt for them as my "ancestors" in Reiki gave way to heartfelt love for them as individuals and enormous gratitude for their comforting presence in my life. Takata began to feel like a grandmother to me, and Hayashi and Usui like grandfather and great-grandfather. When I was in need of guidance, when I was in doubt, when I was hurt by an unkindness I could not comprehend, I could go to them to "talk"— and receive the benefit of their wisdom and the blessing of their love. When I felt faced with a Reiki healing request that challenged my ability to stay centered and calm—sending healing to a friend or family member about to undergo surgery, for example—I could call them in and ask them to be present at the operation to guide the surgeon's hands and to send healing—and the operation would go beautifully.

CHOICES, CHOICES

Once I got into the habit of connecting to Mikao Usui, Chujiro Hayashi, and Hawayo Takata for guidance as I did distant healing, I discovered that so much guidance came I often felt overwhelmed. Again and again I was reminded that I had a wonderful array of spiritual tools to use for self-healing and transformation.

Finally, I asked them if I was meant to apply all this advice. There was so much! No, they said, not at all. I was meant to use my self-knowledge, my discernment, and my free will to choose. Choose one suggestion to apply, or, if I felt I had the commitment to make a greater effort, choose two or three to apply in turn, noticing the individual and cumulative effects on my life.

This guidance greatly lightened my sense of guilt. I appreciate the gift of spiritual insight and encouragement so much; I truly want to value it by acting on it in the appropriate way at the appropriate time. However, by offering lots of help but refusing to recommend one course of action over another, the teachers allow me to remain empowered to make my own choices. They also allow me to grow to realize my highest good, without developing an unhealthy dependence on them for guidance. Finally, by giving me the freedom to choose, the teachers give me permission to be human and just who and what I am—imperfect, committed to improving as a person, as a spiritual being in a physical body, as a soul.

REIKI GUIDANCE TO TEACH

As I continued to do Reiki, to take on more clients and to spend more time each day doing distant healing, I wondered about the void left by my own teacher's retirement. Who would teach Reiki to those who wanted to learn? Over the course of the early 1990s, I heard of one or two of my fellow students who had become Reiki Masters. Good! I thought. At least, there are a couple of people teaching in the Philadelphia area.

Then one night I dreamed about the end of the world. It was not a nightmarish apocalyptic vision; it was heralded with a siren blaring and a voice announcing over a loudspeaker that a hostile foreign country had launched atomic warheads against the United States. Although a counterattack had been launched, landfall of the first warheads was anticipated in fifteen minutes. I stood in a second-floor corridor of a factory building, looking out a window at the panicked civilians below running in all directions. I could hear the muffled shouts of mothers calling their children, see the desperation as frantic husbands searched for their wives and families. Behind me, factory workers pounded through the corridor, rushing to get outside the building, to their cars, to—where? With fifteen minutes to landfall, I knew that no one would escape.

I had fifteen minutes to live. What did I want to do with it? I knew! I turned away from the window and caught the attention of a few of the people running through the corridor. "Sit down," I told them, pointing to a bench below the window. "I want to show you something that is really important." I placed my hands over my lower rib cage. "This is where you place your hands to begin to do a Reiki treatment on yourself."

The alarm clock shrilled, and I woke up, stunned by the message of the dream. I had never thought about teaching Reiki, at least not consciously. I was quite certain that whatever was required of a human being to teach Reiki, I didn't have it. Whatever gentleness and compassion I possessed were offset by countless faults, endless negative thinking, a bottomless well of guilt and shame. How could I ever teach? Yet, if I understood the dream correctly, I was to consider pursuing the master course.

Over the next several months I thought about what this life-long commitment would mean, how it might change me, how it might affect my relationship with my family. Tentatively I began to do some research to locate possible teachers. I talked with several, finally committing to take the Reiki Master course with a woman in New Jersey who would teach it to me over three days. This seemed to be far too little time to "master" anything, but the woman's price was what I could afford. I wrote a check for $100, sent it away as a deposit, and in return the woman sent me her manuals for Reiki I and II and asked me to complete my application by answering a couple of essay questions. Finally, on the weekend before I was to take her class, I studied her manuals and discovered that the way that she used the second Reiki symbol was far more limited than the way I had been trained to use it. In addition, her manual had pages and pages of grounding and centering exercises that were completely unnecessary to doing Reiki. The more that I looked at these exercises, the more I became convinced that this teacher had added information to whatever Reiki training she had been given, devaluing its power. I realized that I did not want this woman to teach me the Reiki master course.

I called her and asked her directly about the additional exercises, and she acknowledged changing the course content from what she had been given. "I'm sorry," I told her. "I don't want to continue my Reiki training with you."

She was angry. "Well, I can't return your deposit, as I've already bought the material for the manual."

"That's all right. I understand. Please keep the deposit," I said. "Good-bye." I hung up the phone with very mixed feelings. If I was to learn Reiki, who could teach me? How could I possibly afford the instruction that I wanted?

In the weeks that followed I mulled these questions over without coming up with a clear answer. I was tempted to call Frank DuGan again. I knew that he had been Beth Gray's student for Reiki I and II, so we would at least have common ground as a starting point. He had also promised to teach me over time, taking as long as necessary to support me through the energetic transformation of the Reiki Master attunement and through the transmittal of the teachings. The price he asked, though, was far beyond what I thought I could afford.

Then one day I reached for a book from my shelf, held it closed in my hands as I said a prayer for guidance, and then opened it up to read these words from the Bible, from the Gospel of Matthew 13:45–46, "The kingdom of heaven is like a merchant seeking beautiful pearls, who, when he had found the one pearl of great price, went and sold all that he had and bought it." I had asked for guidance and now I had an answer. I knew what I must do.

I called Frank DuGan and told him that I wanted to study the Reiki Master course with him, even though I didn't know how I could pay for the course. He was delighted—and agreeable to payment arrangements. He turned out to be the perfect teacher for me for the master course. Although very different from Beth Gray, his love of Reiki was matched by the bold curiosity of a former police investigator. This appealed to me as a researcher and writer. I made the decision to study with Frank DuGan and was certified by him on December 18, 1994.

TAKATA'S LAUGHTER

In early 1996, I sent out my book proposal for *Traditional Reiki for Our Times* to half a dozen publishers and then forgot about it, knowing it would be months before any of the publishers replied one way or another. In May, I moved from the city into an unfinished apartment on the second floor of a house in a beautiful wooded area of Bucks County; I spent the summer laying down linoleum tiles, priming and painting walls and trim, and putting down carpet. As cooler weather turned summer's lush green into a blaze of flaming colors, I moved furniture into place, hung favorite prints and photos on the walls, arranged books for accessibility to my computer and to my Reiki room. In this room I would teach Reiki, treat clients, and write the book manuscript, should I be asked to do so by any willing publisher.

Sitting in this quiet haven, feeling settled at last, I decided to ask the teachers for guidance about the book. Should I simply go ahead and write the rest of it, whether I had heard from a publisher or not? I called in Mikao Usui, Chujiro Hayashi, and Hawayo Takata, wanting to have their joint approval of any further writing efforts I made. I asked my question, waited in silence for a fraction of a second, and then heard Takata's laughter and the words in a female voice: "Just write the book. Just write the book!" When pressed for clarification she would give none, although I heard more laughter and the same words of encouragement.

Feeling not a little frustrated, I thanked the teachers and ended the session. I puzzled over the message all that evening and most of the next day—until the phone call came in the afternoon from the acquisitions editor at Inner Traditions/Healing Arts Press telling me that the company would like to offer me a contract for *Traditional Reiki for Our Times*.

I was delighted—and very grateful; I was also amazed, yet again, at the foresight of the teachers and pleased that they could take pleasure in the prospect of the writing of this book.

Perhaps because I sensed that they were glad to be invited in to help me with my writing, I called upon them again and again as I wrote, often requesting their advice when I wrestled with wording. Because of their willingness to provide guidance to me, page after page, I almost felt that I should credit them as coauthors. Instead, I have simply thanked them in my heart whenever practitioners have contacted me to say that they feel so much Reiki energy in their hands as they read it. That's wonderful, I say. I felt it, too!

MIKAO USUI'S GUIDING HAND

That fall and winter, as I worked steadily to complete the book manuscript for *Traditional Reiki For Our Times*, I connected to Dr. Usui through the Reiki distant-healing method, wanting guidance. Even though I often repeated to myself the Reiki principle, "Just for today, do not worry," I could not shake the sense of anxiety that I felt. How could I possibly write a book that was good enough to honor the great good that Reiki brings into the world? To write a single word that was inaccurate or misleading would feel like a sin or a crime. Yet how could I be certain of the details when research on Reiki in Japan had just barely begun? What if I offended someone unwittingly? What if I violated some sacred trust by writing so comprehensively? These and other anxious thoughts plagued me.

One night I dreamt that I clung to a single branch of a slender young sapling planted on top of a slippery slope of mud up against a high wall. Of course, I felt fearful of falling—and of failing—and the dream let me know that, awake or asleep, my fear had me in its grip. The day after this dream I asked Dr. Usui to help me by showing me how to survive the process of writing the book with my love for Reiki intact. "Please don't use words," I asked him. "My mind is too full of words. Please show me."

And so he did: through distant healing, the first image that he showed me was of his own outstretched hand, a bit browner than mine, with wider, squarer fingers and palm, holding a beautiful, luminous pearl. As I understood what I saw—a personal symbol of Reiki, which had been described to me in earlier guidance as "the pearl of great price"—he lowered his hand, still holding the pearl, into a shallow stream of fast-moving water. As he rested his hand against the rocky bottom, the current swirled grains of sand around the pearl, but the pearl itself did not move. And then his hand became my hand, and I understood what I was to do: I was to go more deeply inside with my practice of Reiki, so that whatever emotional currents or professional criticism swirled about me, my love for Reiki would not be affected in any negative way. I was to focus my intention on the truth of my experiences, honor my guidance to complete the book, and find peace and clarity in my daily practice.

The power of this guidance was so calming, so comforting to me that I cried with gratitude—and found that I was, indeed, able to honor the calling I felt to write *Traditional Reiki for Our Times*.

AN ANIMAL MESSENGER

Shortly after I began to teach Reiki, a practitioner friend introduced me to Ted Andrews' wonderful book, *Animal-Speak*, which includes a comprehensive dictionary of animal, bird, and reptile symbolism. My friend and I experimented with sending Reiki to the same willing client. When intuitive impressions about this client came to her in words and to me in images of animals, we looked in this book together and were delighted to discover that our impressions corresponded.

I bought a copy of the book for myself and began to thumb through its pages to learn more about the historic and cross-cultural symbolism of the animals and birds I glimpsed in the woods around my home. The deer that have always fascinated me with their grace and agility, I learned, are the only creatures who came to hear the Buddha's first sermon, when he finally broke his long silent meditation under the boddhi tree. As I thought about teaching Reiki I recognized that I should be willing to teach with the dedication of the Buddha, simply committed to speaking the truth for anyone willing to learn. As I began to schedule classes, people came to learn Reiki; it was never necessary for me to go out into the woods on a day when I had scheduled a class and test my dedication. Would I be willing to teach with no other human being to hear, to stand in a clearing in the woods and see if blue jays would stop to hear or dragonflies pause in their flight? Such a romantic, impractical notion!

Yet just after I finished my manuscript for *Traditional Reiki for Our Times*, just before dawn on a cool, spring morning, I rubbed at my tired eyes, rose from my desk chair, and stretched. Then I walked into my bedroom to look out my window at the new day. There, in the driveway below my window, was a single deer looking up at me. I watched her for a few minutes as the rising sun began to color the new day with pale gold light. "Thank you," I whispered. "Thank you for the message."

Feeling a depth of gratitude for Reiki and all that I had learned and had yet to learn, I turned away from the window and returned to my office to ready the manuscript for a Federal Express pick up. The next time I looked out the window, the deer had gone.

ENCOURAGING REIKI PRACTITIONERS TO ASK FOR GUIDANCE

After I took my Reiki Master training in 1994 and began to teach, I gradually decided to tell my level II students of the ability we have to connect to the teachers for guidance. This was not something Beth Gray had taught her students, even though she had taught us that we could send Reiki to those who had made their transition. This represented a change in the traditional way I had been taught—and the sharing of a blessing.

On the same foundation of repeated level I and II attunements that I had used since I began to teach, I invited my Reiki II students to practice using distant healing with the method Beth had presented and another much shorter distant-healing method I had learned from Frank DuGan, my teacher for level III. I required them to practice sending Reiki to a client unknown to them, to themselves, and to the world. Finally, I invited them to use the distant healing method to connect to one of the teachers, to offer Reiki healing and to ask for Reiki guidance.

While this is not an easy in-class assignment for a brand new Reiki II practitioner, I continue to require these practice sessions whenever I teach the advanced course. I feel that it is important for every practitioner to know how close at hand the teachers are and how readily they provide help and guidance.

SUGGESTIONS FOR PRACTITIONERS

In the early chapters of this book you were invited to identify how intuition may have guided you on your path to Reiki. Since you have learned Reiki your intuition has continued to guide you in a very personal way, encouraging you to step forward on your spiritual path. Whether or not you have ever attempted to connect through Reiki to Mikao Usui, Chujiro Hayashi, or Hawayo Takata, you may still have experienced being guided about your spiritual path through dreams, through animal messengers, through seeming coincidence, through a knowing without knowing how you knew. Please take the time to remember, and if you are so inclined, to record this important part of your own spiritual history. These memories are not the hidden history of your soul, but that which is on the surface, exposed to your view. These memories are lighted, shining, joyful. Cherish them.

NOW YOU

If you are an advanced Reiki practitioner, you can experiment with connecting to Mikao Usui, Chujiro Hayashi, or Hawayo Takata using the method you were taught. Using the awareness you now have of how intuitive Reiki works, you may simply want to send healing to one of the teachers and say hello—and to see if you get a reply. If you do not receive a reply or any impressions, do not be discouraged. Try again when you feel a little more relaxed and little less anxious. If you are patient, willing to ask, and open to receiving, the teachers will begin to gently guide you.

The simple method of distant healing that was described in chapter 6 will also work for any advanced practitioner. It can be adapted to the purpose of asking for guidance from Mikao Usui, Chujiro Hayashi, or Hawayo Takata by modifying the wording of step 3, still acknowledging free will and higher purpose. You may "offer Reiki healing" and request Reiki healing and guidance from one or more of the ancestral Reiki teachers. When you feel yourself connect, you may simply enjoy the Reiki energy and wait to see what impressions arise, you may invite a dialogue by introducing yourself and asking a question, or you may listen attentively to whatever wisdom the teacher shares. When you feel the flow of energy begin to diminish and your encounter comes to a close, please remember to express your thanks for guidance and for the gift of Reiki.

13

Expanding Practice: Traditional Japanese Techniques

Perhaps the most extraordinary blessing of Reiki in recent years, besides the rapid increase in the number of practitioners worldwide, has been the gift of knowledge offered by the community of Japanese Reiki practitioners and teachers. At the invitation of Canadian, American, and British Reiki Masters Rick Rivard, Tom Rigler, and Andrew Bowling, Japanese Reiki Master Hiroshi Doi, author of the first Japanese Reiki book, *Iyashino Gendai Reiki-ho* (Modern Reiki Method for Healing), traveled to Canada in the summer of 1999 to share information on the history of Reiki and Japanese Reiki techniques. Hiroshi Doi, a member of the Usui Reiki Ryoho Gakkai (the learning society founded by Mikao Usui) has since visited the West several times, acting as a goodwill emissary, offering access to documents that might have eluded Western researchers for years, and providing instruction in techniques that have been used by members of the Usui Reiki Ryoho Gakkai for generations.

Mr. Doi himself acknowledges that there has been a different emphasis in

Reiki practice on each side of the Pacific. In their aspiration to enlightenment the Japanese have historically focused more on techniques of meditation than practitioners in the West, who have focused on techniques of healing. Besides sharing techniques that have been used within the Usui Reiki Gakkai for decades, many of them created by Dr. Usui himself, Mr. Doi also teaches Gendai Reiki, or modern Reiki, which is his synthesis of the two traditions.

Fortunately, Reiki practitioners who attend one of Mr. Doi's workshops or hear him at a conference discover that Reiki is Reiki, East or West. Anyone attuned as a practitioner can learn to do the techniques he presents and enjoy a deepening of the experience of the Reiki energy. There is also sometimes an opportunity to have guidance validated: when I realized that *gassho*, the practice of bringing one's hands together at the heart, was a traditional Japanese technique, I felt a thrill of recognition. For years, before beginning a Reiki treatment I had been making this simple gesture because it brought the Reiki energy very strongly into my hands. At the close of a treatment it seemed natural to bring my hands into this position as well, in gratitude for the power of Reiki and the opportunity of service. I was delighted to discover that the Japanese practitioners begin and end a treatment—and most techniques—with gassho. Though I had been initiated first in the Western tradition, I knew I could feel comfortable learning and teaching traditional Japanese techniques; intuitively, it felt right.

I studied the traditional Japanese Reiki techniques, called Usui Reiki Ryoho, with Reiki Master Tom Rigler of Baltimore, Maryland, one of Hiroshi Doi's sponsors to the West. Tom taught me a wide array of Shoden, Okuden, and Shinpiden techniques in an intensive workshop and then certified me to teach in April 2001. In January 2002, I was instructed in Gendai Reiki by Tom Rigler, who certified me to teach Hiroshi Doi's modern blending of the two traditions. Finally, in late September and early October 2002, I traveled to Toronto, Canada, to attend the fifth Usui Reiki Ryoho International Conference. At this conference I had the pleasure of meeting Mr. Hiroshi Doi and Zen Buddhist priest Hyakuten Inamoto and other Japanese Reiki Masters. I spent time with them in advance of the conference. I attended their presentations with avid interest, which allowed me to review all the traditional Japanese Reiki techniques I had been taught by Tom Rigler and to learn a few that were newly introduced.

The techniques described below are based on the step-by-step instructions given in *Usui Reiki Ryoho: Shoden, Okuden and Shinpiden Japanese Reiki Workshop Manual* by Rick R. Rivard and Tom Rigler. Although many more traditional Japanese techniques are presented within the pages of this manual by Rivard and Rigler, those that follow have been selected because they provide another foundation for the use of intuition in Reiki practice.

Gassho

The technique of joining the hands together at the heart is so simple and natural that it has been used across cultures and across recorded time as a sign of humility, respect, and reverence. In traditional Japanese Reiki, gassho marks the moment of setting one's intention to work with the Reiki energy. A practitioner will bring hands together in gassho at the beginning of a Reiki treatment, and at its close. A Reiki Master will bow to a student, with hands in gassho position, at the start of an attunement; when the attunement is completed, the Master, hands in gassho position, will again bow; the student usually will also gassho and bow.

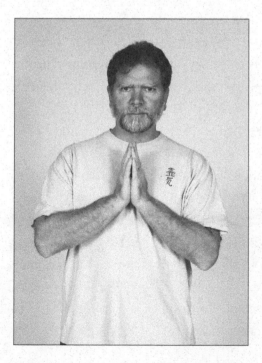

Figure 13.1

1. Sit or stand comfortably, with your eyes open or closed as circumstances require. Allow your heart to fill with your love of Reiki.
2. In respect and reverence, bring your outstretched hands together, palm to palm, at the level of your heart (fig. 13.1). Enjoy the feeling of the Reiki energy that flows into them.

Kenyoko-ho, or Dry Brushing

This technique is used to call for spiritual cleansing and protection. The ritualized brushing off of the torso and arms should be done with the intention of cleansing both the physical body and the energetic body or aura. With a few swipes of our hands we brush away the dust and grime of daily life along with anger, worry, fear, and any other negative thoughts and feelings.

1. Stand tall or sit up straight, breathing in a comfortable, relaxed way. Set your intention to begin this cleansing ritual by saying aloud or in the silence of your mind, "I begin Kenyoko-ho now." (Westerners may feel more comfortable setting their intention in English: "I begin this ritual with the intention of cleansing both my physical body and my energy field.")
2. Place your right hand, fingers extended and straight, on your left shoulder (fig. 13.2). In a quick, sweeping motion, brush your right hand down across your chest until your right arm drops into a relaxed, comfortable position at your side (figs. 13.3 and 13.4).
3. Perform the same action again, this time connecting your left hand to your right shoulder. When you place your left hand on your right shoulder, your fingers should be extended and straight (fig. 13.5). Then in a quick, sweeping motion, brush your left hand down across your chest until your left arm drops into a relaxed position at your side (figs. 13.6 and 13.7).
4. Repeat the brushing of the torso with the right hand to left shoulder, exactly as in step 2. At the end of the motion, allow your right arm to rest naturally at your side.
5. With your right hand, fingers extended, use a quick sweeping motion to brush your left arm from the shoulder down to the wrist (figs. 13.8 and 13.9).

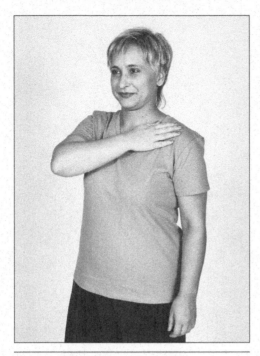

Figure 13.2

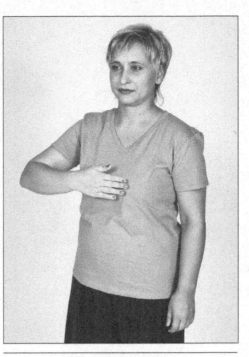

Figure 13.3

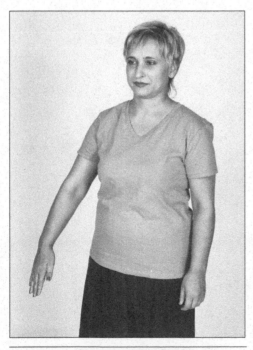

Figure 13.4

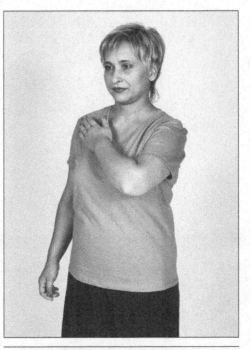

Figure 13.5

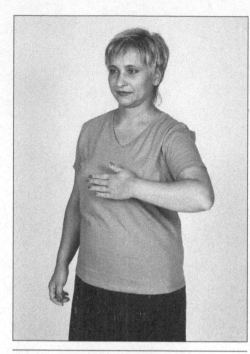

Figure 13.6

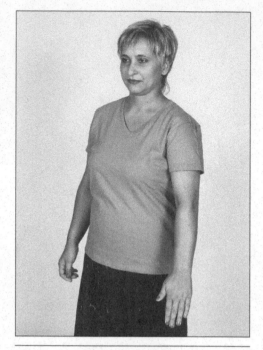

Figure 13.7

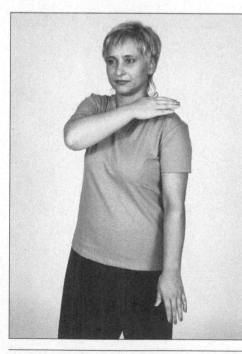

Figure 13.8

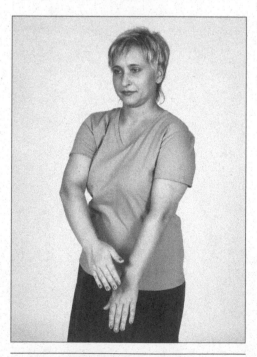

Figure 13.9

(You may discover that it is more comfortable for you to perform this motion if you raise your left arm slightly, so that it extends in front of you.)

6. With your left hand, fingers extended and straight, brush your right arm in a quick sweeping motion from the shoulder down to the wrist (figs. 13.10 and 13.11). (Again, this may be easier to do if you raise your right arm slightly so that it extends in front of you.)

7. Once again, use your right hand to brush your left arm from shoulder to wrist. (Note: the final three strokes may also be made from elbow to wrist, rather than from shoulder to wrist, if this is more comfortable for you.)

8. Relax your arms and hands. You may acknowledge completion of this technique by saying aloud or in the silence of your mind, "I have completed Kenyoko-ho." (Westerners may be more comfortable saying audibly or silently, "I have completed the Reiki cleansing technique.") Then bring your hands together in gassho (fig. 13.12).

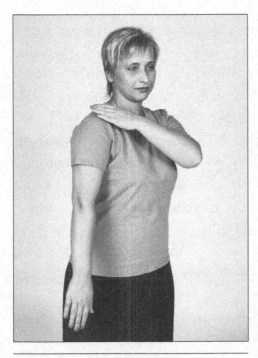
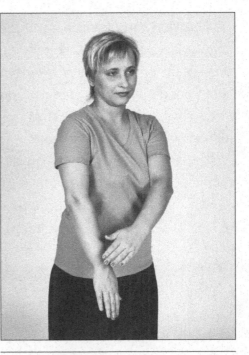

Figure 13.10   *Figure 13.11*

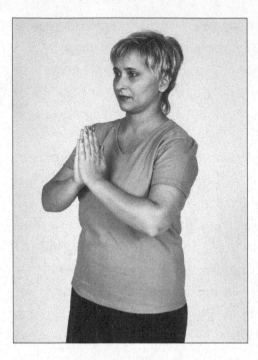

Figure 13.12

When the Japanese perform this technique they do the brush strokes very rapidly. Once you have practiced Kenyoko-ho a bit you will find yourself naturally speeding up as well. Eventually you will be able to perform Kenyoko-ho in a matter of seconds. It is meant to be done quickly, as a preparation for other Reiki practices, such as a meditation or a treatment. Often a practitioner who has performed this technique will move immediately into gassho and then another technique. An alternative way to prepare to do meditation or treatment is to perform Kenyoko-ho, then connect to the Reiki light (described below), and then gassho. Either sequence allows the practitioner to add a level of intention and to express respect for the value of Reiki before beginning extended work with the energy.

Connecting to Reiki Light

Every Reiki Master who has ever lifted his or her hands upward to receive the energy to perform an attunement knows how enlivening this gesture is. Feeling the Reiki energy falling into one's hands and flowing down, into the physical body and mind and into the energy field, is uplifting and empowering.

Making this gesture, whether to prepare for an attunement or a meditation or treatment, invites the Reiki energy into a practitioner's life in the moment. The result is something wonderful.

1. Standing or sitting comfortably, eyes open or closed as circumstances or preference dictates, perform Kenyoko-ho.
2. At the end of the final stroke, raise both arms up high and straight, hands open and fingers extended, as if reaching for the sky (fig. 13.13). Silently or aloud, ask to connect to the Reiki energy and open your awareness to feel it flowing into your hands, down your arms, into your body, into your whole being. Feel yourself surrounded by the Reiki energy, as if you stand in a column of sparkling, swirling, white light.
3. Feeling the Reiki energy flowing through you, feeling gratitude, lower your arms and bring your hands together in gassho.

Note: If you have been taught in the traditional way to listen to the subtle energy in your hands in order to determine when to shift from one hand placement to the

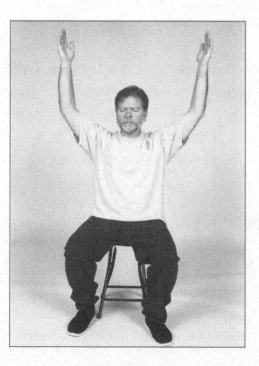

Figure 13.13

next, this technique will be easy. If you have not been taught how to listen to the energy in your hands, accompany the gesture of reaching upward and the request to Spirit to feel the Reiki energy with a visualization of Reiki as a column of white light, humming with current, flowing down from above to you. With your inner eye, see the Reiki energy as a light that fills you and surrounds you with unconditional love and healing. When you are able to imagine yourself radiant with this light, feel your gratitude, and bring your hands into gassho to close. And now you are ready to begin whatever comes next: daily life, meditation, or a Reiki treatment.

Hatsurei-ho, or Cleansing Breathing

This simple, beautiful meditation encourages practitioners to become more aware of the way that Reiki energy comes into them, centers them, and fills them up with healing and peace. In addition, it fosters the awareness that, as Reiki practitioners, we can radiate Reiki energy through every cell. While there are a couple of specific techniques that the Japanese have traditionally taught (radiating Reiki energy through the eyes and through the breath) to employ this awareness in healing, this meditation helps cultivate a consciousness of how to be a healing presence in this world in every moment of every day.

1. Sitting comfortably in a chair or on the floor, close your eyes and relax your arms so that your hands rest gently on your thighs, and focus your awareness on your breath. Consciously relax and begin to slow your breathing. Allow yourself to become aware of your tanden point, located in the middle of the lower abdomen, along the centerline of the body, a few inches below the navel.
2. Set your intention. Aloud or in the silence of your mind say, "I will start Hatsurei-ho now." (Alternately, you might use the words: "I will start the cleansing Reiki meditation now.")
3. Perform Kenyoko-ho, the ritualized dry brushing described above, still with eyes closed, still with a relaxed awareness of your breathing and the tanden point. To deepen the cleansing quality of the ritual you might make a sound as you exhale: "Haaaaaaaah" or "Aaaaaaahhhhhhh." If you feel this audible

breathing (called *hado* breathing by the Japanese) deepens your relaxation, continue to use it during the rest of this meditation.

4. When you have completed Kenyoko-ho, connect to Reiki light (described above) by lifting both arms overhead as high as you can while maintaining a relaxed awareness. Visualize the Reiki energy as light that flows down around you in an energetic column. Feel it flowing around you and into you, filling you up. With this awareness of being in the flow of the Reiki energy, lower your arms down, so that your hands come to rest in your lap.

5. Move your arms so that your hands rest on your thighs. Turn your palms upward so that the fingers are loosely curled and relaxed (fig. 13.14). Breathe slow, deep breaths, in and out from your nose. As you maintain a focus on your breathing and an awareness of your tanden, allow your mind to become calm and clear of all other thoughts.

6. With each breath imagine that you are inhaling Reiki energy through the crown of your head. Let it fill you up and flow throughout your body. Become aware that even your hands and fingers, your feet and toes, feel alive with the Reiki energy.

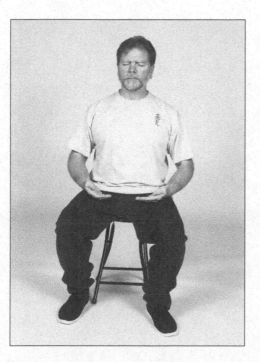

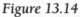

Figure 13.14

7. With each breath, deepen your awareness of the Reiki energy flowing through you. As you inhale, know that you inhale Reiki energy. As you exhale, know that you exhale Reiki energy. Your whole body vibrates with Reiki energy. Feel it radiate out from your skin into the air around you. Know that you are a healing presence in this world.

8. Continue this breathing meditation as long as you like.

9. When you wish to conclude this part of the meditation, simply lift your hands and bring them together in gassho (fig. 13.15).

10. To deepen the meditation even further, practice concentration, called Sei Shin Toitsu. With your hands in gassho, place your awareness on your tanden. Breathe in the Reiki energy, this time visualizing that you are breathing in through your hands into your physical body, down the centerline to the tanden. Allow the Reiki energy to concentrate in the tanden.

11. Breathe out the Reiki energy. Visualize that you are exhaling the Reiki energy you have concentrated in the tanden; exhale it up through the centerline of your body and out through your hands.

12. Continue this Reiki breathing meditation for as long as you like.

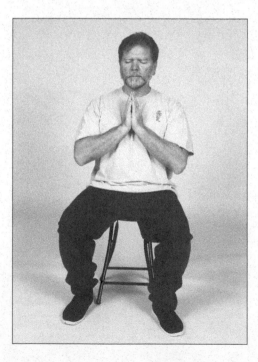

Figure 13.15

13. When you wish to close the meditation, relax your hands and let them come to rest in your lap. Say aloud or in the silence of your mind, "I have completed Hatsurei-ho now." Shake out your hands, blink, look around. Become aware of yourself as a spiritual being in a physical body. Feel your feet on the floor, take in your surroundings.

This meditation is a wonderful way to begin the day; it need not take much time. It can also be used to renew and deepen your sense of connection to the Reiki energy when you feel as if you need to recharge. Regular practice of Hatsurei-ho will enhance your perception of Reiki as subtle energy, for it is another way to "listen to your hands"—as traditionally trained practitioners are taught to do at the bodywork table during client treatments, and during self-treatment.

Meditation on the Reiki Principles

Another good way to begin each day, and to close the day, is to remember the Reiki principles, as Mikao Usui did. This, too, need not take much time, but its impact on the practitioner's sense of connection to Reiki can be profound.

1. Perform Kenyoko-ho.
2. Connect to Reiki light.
3. Gassho.
4. In the silence of your mind or aloud, recite the Reiki principles: "Just for today do not anger; do not worry. Be grateful. Do an honest day's work. Be kind."

Note: if you choose to do the Hatsurei-ho meditation each day, you may close the meditation by reciting the Reiki principles, in speech or in silence, while your hands are still in gassho, then shake out your hands. (According to the Japanese, Mikao Usui would guide his students through this meditation and close with three recitations of the Reiki principles: first, he would say the principles aloud, as the teacher who gives the example; then his students would say them aloud as a group; then each student would say them silently. Sometimes the teacher would then do an attunement.)

Remembering the Reiki principles helps us to choose those courses of action that are for our highest good. They may help us to choose to exercise or to have a piece of chocolate (to be kind to ourselves), to share a crust of bread with a bird or to give a sandwich to a homeless person we meet on the street (to be kind to another), to say a prayer of thanks when we find a convenient parking space or hear the news that progress has been made on an important state or national issue (to practice gratitude). Or they may help us make more difficult choices: to avoid anger the Reiki principles may encourage us not to confront a trespasser, challenge a competitor, make an enemy. When we remind ourselves of the Reiki principles on a regular basis they remain in our awareness, guiding us so that we can live with greater inner peace and enjoyment of life.

Reiki Shower no Giho, or Reiki Shower

The Reiki Shower is not traditional; it is a modern technique taught by Hiroshi Doi as part of Gendai Reiki-ho (modern Reiki method), which combines elements of both the Western and Japanese Reiki traditions in which Mr. Doi is trained. The technique can be used for spiritual cleansing, especially of the aura or energy field. (Note: While it is possible to do this technique seated or standing, it is more comfortable to perform it standing.)

1. Stand or sit in a comfortable posture, feet shoulder-width apart, shoulders relaxed, eyes open or closed, as you prefer.
2. Gassho (fig. 13.16).
3. Connect to Reiki light. With your hands reaching up above you, feel the Reiki flowing down into you, onto you, around you (fig. 13.17). Visualize the flow of Reiki like rainwater showering you with a fine mist of droplets that wash away all that is negative.
4. As you sense the cleansing and healing effects of the Reiki energy, slowly lower your hands to focus in the energy field around your head (fig. 13.18), your neck, your chest and shoulders (fig. 13.19), and down the front of your body (fig. 13.20).

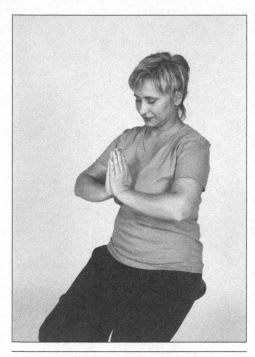

Figure 13.16

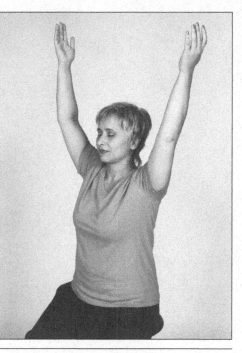

Figure 13.17

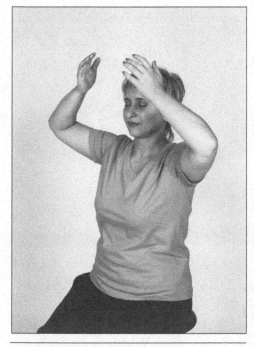

Figure 13.18

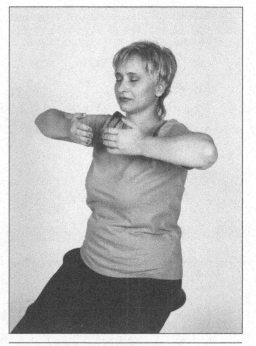

Figure 13.19

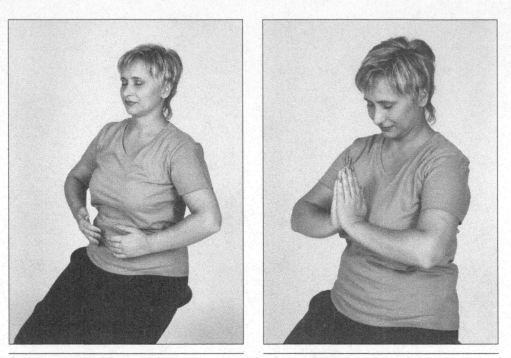

Figure 13.20   *Figure 13.21*

5. If you like the sensation, you may raise your hands up again into the Reiki flow and draw it down again, this time slowly lowering your hands into the energy field at the back of your head, your neck, your shoulders, and down your arms.

6. Repeat this drawing down of the energy into your energy field until you feel that it is clear and clean and vibrant with Reiki. Know that whatever is cleared from your energy is dissolved into light or drawn down through your feet into the earth.

7. Gassho, feeling your gratitude (fig. 13.21).

8. Shake out your hands.

Note: Advanced Reiki practitioners may want to experiment with chanting and/ or visualizing the first symbol as they practice this technique; Reiki Masters may chant or visualize the fourth symbol to enhance the cleansing and healing that occurs.

Just as taking a shower is a sensual pleasure and a sensible hygiene practice for our physical bodies, so too this technique feels good and provides spiritual cleansing. Some practitioners may prefer it to Kenyoko-ho, which serves the same purpose; however, Kenyoko-ho seems more appropriate for professional client treatment and public gatherings, such as Reikishares. When working on oneself the practitioner may want to combine the two, a Reiki shower followed by Kenyoko-ho, to bring the deepest possible cleansing, healing, and recharging to the physical body and the energy field.

Byosen Reikan-ho, or Scanning

As you may have noticed, most of the techniques described so far in one way or another enhance your awareness of Reiki as subtle energy that flows into and through you, not only into your hands but also through your whole physical body and through your energy field. This awareness is very helpful in using Reiki to sense intuitive impressions, for they arise in the same flow of subtle energy; and they become more easily perceptible to you when you have trained yourself to notice variations in energy flow.

Practitioners who are taught traditionally, in the West and most of the world, learn to focus constant, relaxed attention on the sensations in their hands in order to mark the rise, the steady flow, and the ebbing of the Reiki energy. With practice, the level of attention required becomes automatic, making it possible for the practitioner to hold a conversation with the client, listen to background music, and so on. This fundamental skill enables the practitioner to know that the client has received sufficient universal life-force energy in the area under the hands to begin accelerated healing; only after this energetic cycle is complete does the practitioner move on to the next position.

In the West, practitioners are not given any particular name for the expanded range of sensations they experience in their hands when they are doing Reiki on themselves or on a client. They may be told that most new practitioners experience changes in temperature or tingling in their hands as their first sensations of the Reiki flow. With practice they are likely to perceive many more sensations, indicative of the flow of Reiki energy and of the expansion of their perception of that energy. Practitioners describe energy flow in various ways: pulsing; wave-like; whirling; changing in temperature; prickling, like pins-and-needles sensation without the pain. They mention a sense of being held in place (pressure) from above: a sense of being held in place (magnetized) from below; a suction from below; a ray of energy like laser beams shooting off a finger or a part of the palm. The variety of sensations practitioners (and clients) experience at the Reiki table is fascinating; practitioners appreciate the subtlety and complexity, while clients, less focused on specific sensations, enjoy the relaxation and deep healing. There is something so attractive, so comforting and familiar, about this flow of unconditional love that practitioner and clients both keep coming back for more!

In Japan practitioners who are traditionally taught are instructed to notice hibiki (translated as "resonance") in their hands. Here is how Mr. Hiroshi Doi describes hibiki (as translated by Yukio Miura):

> When a person has a disease, you can feel "something" transmitted from the source of the disease. This is called *byosen*. What you feel as byosen varies depending on the type, severity and status of the disease, and from person to person. But some samples are: sensations of something moving, pulsating, or piercing, or of a bug crawling, biting or of pain, numbness, heat, coldness, tickling, tingling, etc.
>
> The sensation you have in your hands is called "hibiki" or "resonance" and by it you can learn to judge the cause of the disease, the status of it and the time it will take to heal.
>
> As long as a person has a disease (even if the person is not aware of it), there never fails to be a byosen. So if you are careful enough to detect the byosen, it is possible to treat the disease a couple of days before it actually shows up. Also there could be a byosen in people who are said to have recovered completely from his/her disease. If you get rid of the byosen in these cases, you can prevent the disease from developing again.
>
> A byosen could show up in the obvious problem area but also could be sensed in areas different from the problem area. For example, the byosen

for stomach disease often shows up in one's forehead; for roundworm it can show up under one's nose; for liver problems it can show up in the eyes, etc.*

Is the instruction to "listen to your hands," given by traditional Usui Reiki Masters to their students in the West, and the instruction to notice the hibiki or resonance in the hands, given by traditional Japanese Reiki Masters to their students the same message? I believe so, although my Usui Reiki Ryoho teacher, Reiki Master Tom Rigler, and I have gone back and forth in conversation, debating this. The ability to listen to the sensations in your hands activated by the flow of Reiki energy for healing is a result of being attuned to Reiki, West or East. The consequence of "listening to your hands" as the energy rises, flows, and ebbs over each area of the body is healing, just as the result of holding hands vibrating with resonance over diseased areas of the body is healing.

Here are a few important differences. In the West, practitioners are taught to apply Reiki-charged hands in each position at least until the first shift in energy before moving to another position; hands are applied in a standard pattern that covers most of the major organs and systems of the body; among the many hand sensations that may arise, pain or discomfort is refused as unnecessary (the practitioner requests that the information that might be conveyed by such sensations be intuitively communicated in another way); the purpose of applying Reiki-charged hands is healing.

In Japan, practitioners are taught to apply Reiki-attuned hands at first using a few standard positions on the head; then, as their sensitivity to the energy becomes greater, they are taught to scan the body slowly and to pause wherever they notice hibiki, or resonance—for beneath their hands is some area of the physical body or energy field that holds evidence of disease. Practitioners maintain their hands over diseased areas until they become quiet and the hand sensations cease. Then they continue scanning until they discover the next area to be treated and repeat the process. The purpose of the treatment is healing.

---

*Hiroshi Doi, quoted in Usui Reiki Ryoho: Shoden, Okuden and Shinpiden Japanese Reiki Workshop Manual by Rick R. Rivard and Tom Rigler, p. 18.

Years ago Japan passed a license-to-touch law. From that time since, all Japanese practitioners have worked primarily in the energy field, floating their hands over the body, to do Reiki client treatments. In the West, traditionally taught practitioners still learn Reiki (in level I) as a hands-on healing method; with more experience and advanced instruction, they, too, often come to recognize the value of applying Reiki-attuned hands not only to the physical body but to the energy field as well.

The energy field is less dense and allows Reiki to move quickly; it holds habitual thoughts and feelings, including negative ones that may need healing; it holds potential disease conditions, not yet manifested in the body, that can be treated and resolved before becoming manifest. The energy field, treated after hands-on treatment of the physical body, acts like a protective shield, enabling the client to enjoy the healing benefits of the hands-on Reiki treatment for a longer period of time.

Learning the practice of Byosen Reikan-ho will allow you to experience and appreciate all of these aspects of the energy field that surrounds the human body. Just as it is not necessary to know human anatomy in order to do Reiki, neither is it necessary to know energy anatomy in order to do this traditional Japanese Reiki technique. If you are acquainted with the chakras or the energy meridians or the layers of the aura, you may find yourself noticing these in the energy field. This is fine, but let your primary purpose be to notice those areas of the body that need healing and apply your hands to accomplish that purpose.

1. Make sure that your client is comfortable, either sitting in a chair or laying on a bodywork table.
2. Perform Kenyoko-ho, or Dry Brushing, to cleanse your own energy field.
3. Connect to Reiki light, extending both arms up to invite Reiki energy to flow into you and through you.
4. Gassho.
5. Approach the client with gentleness, your arms slightly raised, your hands outstretched.
6. Starting over the client's head, place your hands in the client's energy field, floating your hands above the body at whatever level you notice sensations in your hands (fig. 13.22). It is fine to raise and lower your hands slowly

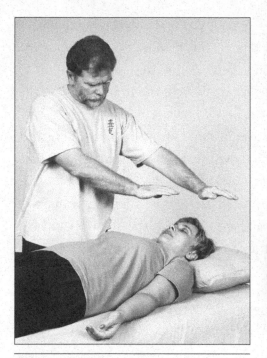

Figure 13.22

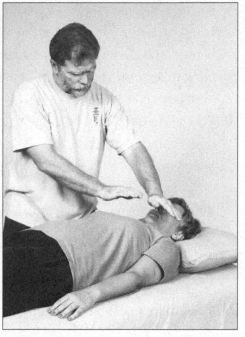

Figure 13.23

in the field until you find the level that you notice the most sensations (where you feel the most hibiki, or resonance).

7. Staying at this level above the client's body, move slowly downward, as if tracing an outline (fig. 13.23).

8. Wherever you notice the hibiki, the hand sensations, increase or intensify, stop to treat the client with Reiki (fig. 13.24). Honor the energy by staying in this position as the energy rises (the hibiki becomes more noticeable), flows steadily (the hibiki stays at the same level of intensity), then subsides (the hibiki

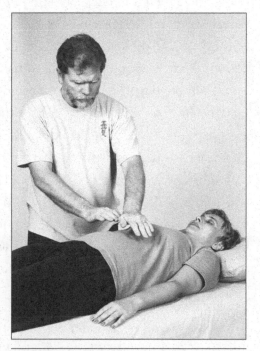

Figure 13.24

becomes quieter, calmer, fades away). Even if you find yourself holding your hands in each position for an extended time (which will vary according to the byosen in the area beneath your hands), be willing to stay: you will be delivering exactly the right "dosage" of Reiki energy medicine to best support the client's healing.

9. When you have finished treating an area, resume scanning. You are finished when your hands remain quiet as you move them slowly through the client's energy field, from over the top of the head to the soles of the feet.

10. Gassho, closing the Reiki treatment. Shake out your hands and arms. Say the client's name softly or touch the client gently on the shoulder to help the client understand that the treatment is over and it is time to return to conscious awareness.

Reiji-ho, or Intuitive Placement of Hands

This is the technique that Hawayo Takata regarded as one of the great secrets of Reiki, as she noted in her diary entry of May 1936: "Mr. Hayashi has granted to bestow on me . . . Leiji-Ho—the utmost secret in the Energy Science." Indeed, learning how to do Reiji-ho makes a practitioner intensely aware that Reiki originates in Source or Spirit, and the connection to Reiki Energy is a connection to Spirit. Although a practitioner may come to understand much about the nature of Reiki healing through practice, Source (or Spirit or God) remains a beautiful and awe-inspiring mystery. Takata knew this. Reiki Master Beth Gray, Takata's beloved friend and student and my teacher for the basic and advanced course, told us that Takata would sometimes admit, "Reiki power, God power." This awareness and acknowledgment encourages the practitioner to more consciously pursue spiritual pathwork. This technique requires that the practitioner go to Spirit step by step by step. To seek guidance in this way, over and over again, in order to complete a Reiki treatment is a wonderfully healing, and humbling, experience.

1. Have your client lie face up on a bodywork table. Offer a pillow to support the head and neck and a pillow or bolster to support the legs under knees. Make sure the client feels comfortable.

2. Perform Kenyoko-ho, or Dry Brushing, to cleanse your own energy field.

3. Connect to Reiki light, extending both arms up to invite Reiki energy to flow into you and through you.

4. Gassho (fig. 13.25).

5. Set your intention to perform a Reiki treatment using Reiji-ho. You might say to yourself, "I will begin Reiji-ho now."

6. Holding your hands in the gassho position, raise them up to your forehead (fig. 13.26). Lightly touch your hands in gassho against the center of your forehead, just above your eyebrows (the area of the sixth chakra, the seat of intuition, according to Indian models of energy anatomy). For most practitioners the information you desire to be guided by will come more easily if you close your eyes as you treat your client, so that all external distractions are shut out.

7. Ask the Reiki energy to show you where to begin the Reiki treatment. Be open to receiving this information as an image, a word, a tactile sensation, a knowing without knowing how you know. (When I do Reiji-ho, the

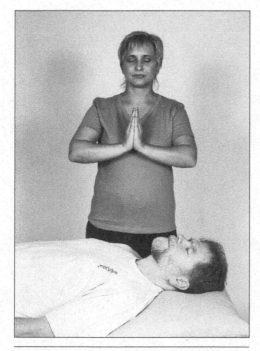

Figure 13.25

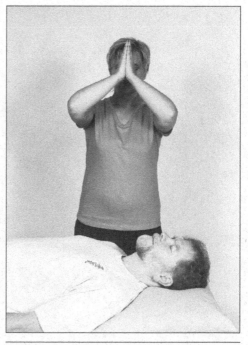

Figure 13.26

information often comes as a kind of color overlay over the area of the client's body that I am to treat next. Sometimes the colors are bright and clear; sometimes they are murky. Either way, if an area is highlighted with color, I treat that area next.) Be patient if the information doesn't come immediately. Hold your hands in gassho to your forehead until the intuitive impression comes.

8. When you have received the guidance you seek, lower your hands from the gassho position and separate them. Approach the client with a quiet mind, a peaceful heart, your Reiki-charged hands outstretched.

9. Place your hands down gently, lightly, over the area of the client's body that you were shown by the Reiki energy (fig. 13.27). If the area in need is one normally considered private, do not place your hands down, but simply place them in the energy field above that area.

10. Allow your hands to remain in position through at least one cycle of the Reiki energy—a gradual or sudden increase in hand sensations, which rises to become a steady level of hand sensations for some period of time (deter-

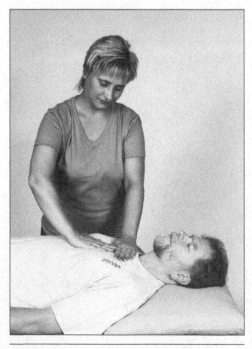

Figure 13.27

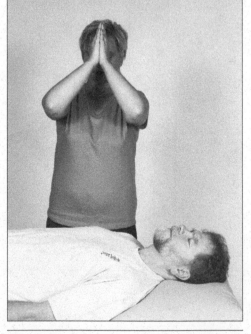

Figure 13.28

mined by the client's byosen, or need for healing), and then just as gradually or suddenly decreases.

11. Step back from the client, bring your hands into gassho, close your eyes, feel the Reiki energy. Raise your hands, in gassho, up to touch the center of your forehead, and ask the Reiki energy to show you the next area of the client's body that you are to treat (fig. 13.28).

12. When you have received the information as an intuitive impression or knowing, lower your hands, and move around the table as necessary to treat the client as you have been directed by the Reiki energy.

13. Again, apply your Reiki-charged hands over this area of the client's body through at least one cycle of the energy (fig. 13.29).

14. When you have completed treatment of this area of the client's body, step back from the table and repeat the process of bringing your hands into gassho, raising them in gassho to your forehead, and asking the Reiki energy for guidance.

15. In this way treat the client until you receive guidance from the Reiki energy that the Reiki treatment is done.

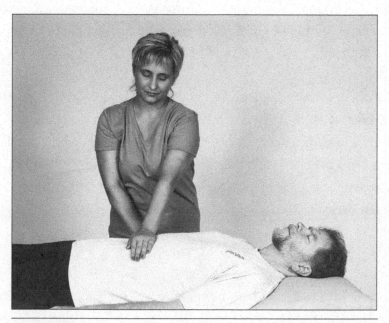

Figure 13.29

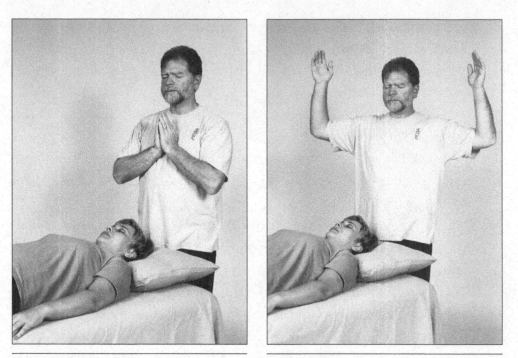

Figure 13.30   **Figure 13.31**

16. Gassho, feeling gratitude in your heart that you are able to connect to the Reiki energy in this way and give Reiki with such guidance to your clients. Say to yourself, "I have completed Reiji-ho now," to indicate that you have fulfilled your intention.

17. Shake out your hands and arms. Let your client know the treatment is concluded by saying the client's name softly or touching the client gently on the shoulder. Encourage the client to return to normal awareness slowly and gently. Help the client, as needed, to sit up and get down from the table.

18. An alternate way to ask for guidance from the Reiki energy is simply to raise your hands, as if connecting to Reiki light, rather than raising your hands in gassho to your forehead (figs. 13.30, 13.31, and 13.32).

This traditional Japanese Reiki technique is a beautiful demonstration that intuition works in complete harmony with the healing purpose of Reiki. Repeated practice of this technique fosters enhanced intuition in every area of

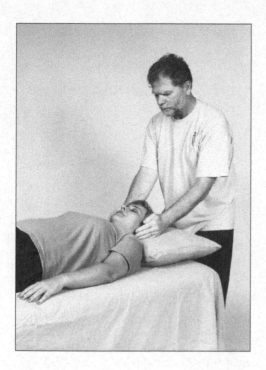

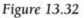

Figure 13.32

the practitioner's life. Notice, however, that in order for the technique to work effectively the practitioner must ask, again and again, for Reiki guidance. Ask and you shall receive. This great spiritual lesson, one that is emphasized across religions, is offered again here.

SUGGESTIONS FOR PRACTITIONERS

Be open to learning about Reiki, as it is practiced in other lineages, at all levels. Do not discard caution, but do allow yourself to be guided to learn that which feels right to you. Do ask to be guided to learn only that which is for your highest spiritual good.

Understand that the true teacher of Reiki, in all its variations, is Reiki itself. Do not become so attached to a particular human teacher or teaching tradition or lineage that you limit your own spiritual growth. Be wary of human teachers who ask you to promise never to go outside their lineage to learn Reiki. This is not empowering to you; it is wholly disempowering. Trust Reiki. Remember the

Reiki principle "Just for today, do not worry," and allow yourself to follow your own inner guidance.

NOW YOU

This entire chapter is an invitation to you to experiment with the traditional Japanese techniques described. Please do experiment first with those techniques that are to be performed individually, especially the Reiki cleansing breath meditation, Hatsurei-ho.

Once you feel comfortable with these techniques, ask a Reiki practitioner friend to be your first client for a practice session using Byosen-ho, and then another using Reiji-ho. After each session be sure to ask your client for feedback on how receiving Reiki feels when the treatment is performed in this way. When you feel comfortable and confident that you can perform these techniques effectively, consider integrating them into your professional client practice. If you are a Reiki Master and you find these techniques effective and enjoyable, please consider learning all the techniques that the traditional Japanese Reiki Masters have shared by seeking out a certified teacher of Usui Reiki Ryoho to teach you Shoden, Okuden, and Shinpiden.

14

EXPANDING PRACTICE: AT A REIKI AND INTUITION WORKSHOP

Over the course of a weekend, advanced Reiki practitioners and teachers of different lineages, both traditional and nontraditional, come together in the spirit of community to practice the healing skill of intuitive Reiki. In a typical workshop we begin by sitting in a circle and joining in a brief meditation, similar to the Japanese technique of "connecting to Reiki light."

☙ ❧

Make yourself comfortable. Let your hands rest naturally in your lap, nested together against your abdomen, or let them drop down and rest easily against your thighs. Notice as the Reiki energy begins to flow through your hands.

Now close your eyes. Become more aware of your breathing. Notice each inhalation and exhalation; consciously slow your breathing. Let yourself relax more deeply. Feel the Reiki energy circulating through your entire body.

Focus again on your breath. Notice how each long, slow breath rises and falls right through your center, up and down along the column of your spine. With this awareness of your center and the Reiki energy gently radiating through your whole body, imagine that you sit in a column of white light that extends infinitely high above you and infinitely far below, grounding in the earth. Imagine that this light is Reiki light, universal life-force energy. Imagine that you can breathe in Reiki light through the crown of your head.

Take a deep, slow breath, drawing in Reiki light through the crown of your head. Feel that breath fill you and flow into your core and radiate out, all the way down your arms to your hands, all the way down your legs to the soles of your feet.

With every breath inhale Reiki light, exhale Reiki light. With every breath become filled with Reiki light, and as you exhale, radiate Reiki light. Continue to breathe in Reiki light, breathe out Reiki light for as long as you like. Let yourself relax deeply in the flow of the energy. Let yourself become radiant, shimmering with Reiki light.

Allow yourself to remember the Reiki principles. Recite them in the silence of your own mind: "Just for today, do not anger . . . do not worry . . . be grateful . . . do an honest day's work . . . be kind." Continue to breathe in Reiki light through the crown of your head, and breathe out Reiki light, radiating it from every cell in your body.

Whenever you are ready to return to more ordinary awareness, bring your hands together, palm to palm, at your heart. Slowly open your eyes.

☙ ❧

After some stretches and yawns and smiles, we spend a few minutes discussing our experiences, then I remind the group of our purpose: we are here to practice intuitive Reiki techniques, to become more confident of our abilities, more comfortable in presenting impressions to clients. We are here to learn how to recognize and honor our inner guidance.

Since stories have the power to raise awareness and to invite considered change, we turn to storytelling. I ask all those in the circle to introduce themselves and to share some aspect of their journey to Reiki. Some are able to recall a coincidence, an intuitive impulse, something that prompted them to learn Reiki.

"My girlfriend mentioned that she was going to take a Reiki class at a church nearby and I told her that I wanted to take the class too, even though I had never heard of Reiki."

"I was in a bookstore, just browsing, and this one book caught my attention. When I picked it up and opened it, my hands just came alive. I felt heat and tingling and pulsing. I thought, 'Wow! I'd better read this book'—and, of course, it was about Reiki."

"I can't say that there was anything in particular that led me to Reiki. I'm in massage school, so I hear about a lot of adjunct therapies. When I heard that there would be a Reiki class offered one weekend during the semester, I felt that I should take it. It just seemed like a good idea."

"I was offered a Reiki treatment by my cousin. It was amazing! I'd had a really stressful day at work, and as soon as I got on her table and she started working on me, I relaxed. I wanted to be able to do that for myself and my family. So I asked her about Reiki classes. That's how I started."

"I have a strange story. I went to a psychic and she told me that I would really enjoy being involved in some form of hands-on healing. 'You have healing hands,' she said. She told me that I might like Reiki. Later that week I saw an ad for a class on the bulletin board at the health food store near where I live. I took the Reiki I class and I loved it. Soon after, I took Reiki II—and now here I am."

"So it seems," I observe, "that some of you have experienced intuition on your way to Reiki, and some of you experienced Reiki directly or researched it, and that motivated you to learn Reiki." Heads nod in response.

"It's interesting how intuition works, isn't it? One of you knew you wanted to learn Reiki without knowing how you knew. One of you was drawn to a book—guided by some inner awareness—and then, when you picked up the book, you had sensations of energy in your hands. And you"—I look toward the woman who visited a psychic—"are open to being guided by your intuition, and you honor the ability in others.

"Just from what we've shared here, it's easy to see that intuition can guide us in different ways. *Intuition* is a very broad term, isn't it? My teacher for Reiki I and II, Beth Gray, told us that just as we have five senses for perceiving the external world, intuition is more than just a 'sixth sense,' because it offers us an equivalent set of inner senses—and more. Probably the easiest to understand is inner vision. We can see with our inner eye—what yogis call the 'third eye' or spiritual eye—dreams, daydreams, memories, and imagined realities, like the window display that we have designed and are assembling at work, or the dinner that we are planning to cook for our guests at Thanksgiving, or the world inhabited by characters in a book. Almost everyone has this ability to see with the inner eye.

"You may have heard the term *clairvoyant,* used to describe people who are gifted with an ability to see with the inner eye events in the future, in the distant past, or across a physical space. *Clairvoyant* is a French word that has made its way into our language unchanged; it means 'clear seeing.' Some of you may already have had experiences with 'clear seeing' as you did Reiki on a client or on yourself, in which you glimpsed images from the future, the past, or from another location.

"The French gave us a few other words that are useful in understanding intuition: *deja vu,* which means 'already seen.' This describes the momentary awareness that people sometimes have that they have already seen or experienced something. Another term is *clairaudience,* used to name the ability to hear clearly with the inner ear—voices not in the room or voices at a distance. Another word, *clairsentience,* describes an inner knowing. These three inner senses—clear seeing, hearing, and knowing—seem to be more common than the inner awareness of a smell, a taste, or a touch, but many people have experienced these forms of intuition too. Sometimes, intuition seems to work best when we are inwardly focused, as we so often are when we do Reiki, but intuition can also come to us as an awareness superimposed over ordinary reality."

One of the practitioners volunteers that she has the ability to know when a friend is thinking of her because she notices a scent she associates with her friend. She has checked back with her friend and so far has never been wrong in this awareness.

"Do you realize that the story of Hawayo Takata's journey to Reiki gives us an example of clairaudience? Do you recall that she heard an inner voice as she lay, awaiting surgery, and that the voice spoke to her three times, telling her that she didn't need this operation—there was another way?

"So Hawaya Takata is an example of someone who was guided by intuition to learn Reiki. Takata later taught intuitive Reiki techniques to a few of the Reiki Masters she initiated. Intuitive Reiki techniques have also been used in Japan for generations. These techniques are part of what we will be learning during the workshop.

"First, let's share some more stories. Let's see if you can remember your very first experience with intuition, and your response to it. Did you feel good about it? Did you tell anyone about it? How did this person react? Did you feel supported or dismissed? Or did the experience frighten you? Did you resist it or deny it? Were you open to it or did it make you want to shut down? Let's just close our eyes again and take a few minutes to reflect and remember. You may want to jot down some notes as you do this review."

We continue sharing stories for the next few hours, learning about the varieties of intuition by hearing one another describe them. We also learn how important the initial support we received—or didn't receive—was in shaping our later responses to intuition. We explore the role of our families, our churches, our communities, and our culture in helping us feel a level of acceptance for intuition or in making us feel outcast, different, strange. The goal of our storytelling is to begin to become aware of our fears and doubts, and to let them go. While this process is not likely to be completed within the time allotted to the workshop, a good start on it can be made.

How can we heal the wounded self, discouraged from claiming the spiritual gift of intuition by the harsh criticism of a family member or the emotional distancing of a friend? How can we get past the finger-pointing of school children who saw us as "different" at an age when all we wanted was to fit in? How can we learn to trust our own ability to be guided by an inner wisdom when we were brought up within a church community that sternly rejected "false prophets"?

Reiki, which heals on all levels, can heal these spiritual hurts as well. We can use Reiki distant healing to heal our intuition, to free ourselves of self-doubt and fear, to release ourselves from the emotional trauma of the past. We can send

Reiki to the third eye, to the pineal gland, to our conscious connection to our souls. Sometimes very quickly, sometimes more gradually, we will receive the healing for which we ask.

This is, in part, because intuition is a natural ability that is enhanced by Reiki, that supports Reiki and that supports our further spiritual development. This is also, in part, because we do ask—and being willing to ask Spirit for help to accomplish something, if it is for the highest good, is a request that Spirit is unlikely to refuse.

We can also claim healing by educating ourselves about intuition and the purposes it serves. As we understand how integral intuition is to the human experience, we can make a place for it in our lives and recognize it as the guiding impulse of our souls and our hearts.

USING A PENDULUM

Just before we take a mid-day break, I give each student a pendulum. "Reach in and take one," I say, as I send a brown paper bag around the circle. Inside there is a variety of pendulums of carved and polished stone, crystal, and wood, each attached to a simple chain or string.

"You do *not* need a pendulum to do Reiki," I say immediately. "You are already attuned to Reiki and your hands are sensitive to the Reiki energy. Your hands are the only 'physical' tools you need. You do not need props of any kind."

"What about using a pendulum to balance the chakras?" one student asks. "My teacher showed us how to do that in my Reiki II class."

"Just use your hands. Place one hand in the energy field over the heart and the other over the throat, and then the third eye, until the upper chakras are balanced against the heart. Then do the same with the lower chakras. Hold one hand in the energy field over the heart and the other over the solar plexus, then the spleen chakra, then the root chakra. Wait until the energy activity from each chakra feels about the same as the energy activity above the heart. That's an easy way to balance the chakras.

"I hope that you realize that chakra balancing is not part of traditional Usui

Reiki, Western or Japanese. The concept of the chakras comes out of Indian yogic philosophy, which offers us one model of energy anatomy. Oriental medicine offers us another: energy meridians. Both have a value, and yet I would rather not be limited by either one. I would rather listen to my hands in the energy field so that I can sense what needs balance and what needs strengthening and healing. Chakra balancing, in a Reiki class, is a modern addition, not a traditional technique. I think that using a pendulum to do chakra balancing could be really alarming to a client who expects Reiki healing, pure and simple."

"So why are you giving us pendulums," one student asks, "if you have such strong objections to using them with Reiki?"

"Pendulums are a simple way to practice asking for intuitive guidance. The more that you ask for inner guidance, the more you are likely to receive. So using a pendulum can help you to develop the habit. Eventually, though, you want to get to a point in your own spiritual evolution where you don't need a pendulum. You can just close your eyes, take a moment to get centered and grounded, breathe in Reiki energy through the crown of your head, and ask for—and receive—inner guidance that you can trust."

"So how do you use the pendulum?" one student asks.

"I stand or sit in such a way that the pendulum can drop straight down. Then I ask, 'Mother-Father God, will you please guide this pendulum?' If the pendulum moves—and it usually does—I then ask, 'Would you please show me "yes"?'. I wait to see how the pendulum moves. Then I ask, 'Would you please show me "no"?'. Again, I wait to see how the pendulum moves. When those movements are clear, I ask my question, which should be phrased in such a way that it can be answered with a clear 'yes' or 'no.' For me, a straight back-and-forth motion is usually 'yes' and a straight side-to-side motion is usually 'no.' If the pendulum circles, I consider that a 'maybe.'"

"Is it always accurate?"

"It is usually accurate, but just as we can visualize something we are worried about being played out before our inner eye, so we can also project our fears and anxieties into this process. If I suspect that I am doing that, I will ask another question: 'Is this answer a projection of my fears and worries?' If I get a 'yes,' I will ask again, 'Mother-Father God, would you please guide this pendulum?' or I will simply put the pendulum away until I am more relaxed and less anxious."

"Do we have to use that wording? 'Mother-Father God'?"

"No, but I would recommend that you go to the highest source of guidance you recognize. For some of you that will be Christ Consciousness. For others that will be Allah or Jehovah. If you are someone who doesn't believe in God, by any name, you might ask to be guided by your own High Self, your own inborn source of wisdom."

"Why not ask to be guided by someone who has expertise in the area of your question—like Einstein or Martin Luther King?"

"Despite their genius, Einstein and Martin Luther King were also human beings with personalities and preferences and faults of their own. Do you really want to allow yourself to be guided by anyone who is biased or flawed? Go to Source, whatever you call Source. You want to become practiced in going to the highest possible source of wisdom."

At this point most of the students have begun to play with the pendulums they have received. "Playing" is a fair word to use, because this is a gentle, child-like way to interact with Spirit and to learn how to calm yourself enough to ask for clear guidance. After they have had the opportunity to learn the process and to ask a question or two, I remind them to say a silent thank you.

Then I offer a final caution: "Remember that a pendulum is not meant to become a crutch. Your guidance is always available to you, within you, if you are calm enough, clear enough, and remember to ask Spirit. The pendulum is a useful tool to confirm what you already intuitively know. Don't become overly reliant on it. If you do, you will probably lose your pendulum for a while—Spirit's gentle reminder that the answers you need to know are already within you and available to you now, if you are meant to know them at this time.

A Method for Working with a Pendulum

1. Breathe a centering breath of white light, imagining you can inhale through the top of your head and fill up not only your lungs but your whole body, all the way down to the soles of your feet and even below your feet. Breathe in

to relax, calm, ground, and center yourself. Breathe in to invite Spirit to fill you and your energy field with white light.

2. Hold your pendulum in one hand so that it drops straight down (fig. 14.1). Now ask the pendulum if it is willing to be guided by Mother-Father God, Christ, or whatever source of universal life force you acknowledge. (If you prefer you may ask if the pendulum is willing to be guided by your High Self, the source of your highest wisdom.)

3. Mentally ask, "Please show me 'yes.'" Then wait to see what motion is indicated.

4. Mentally ask, "Please show me 'no.'" Again, wait to see what motion is indicated.

5. Get your question clear in your mind, in a form that can be answered with a simple "yes" or "no." For example, you might ask, "Is it for my highest good to take this class in spiritual development?" A question that clearly phrased should result in a clear "yes" or "no" answer. However, you might have multiple opportunities to take the class you are considering. So you might want

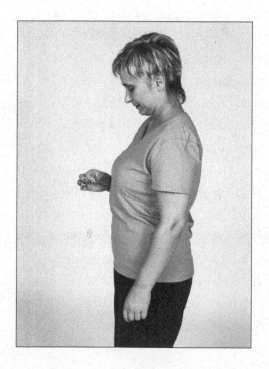

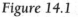

Figure 14.1

to ask another question: "Is it for my highest good to take this class on the weekend of April 12th and 13th this year?" If you get another affirmative, you have a pretty good indication that you should go ahead and take the class. If your pendulum circles or wobbles, you have a "maybe." Ask your question in another way for more clarification.

6. Remember to thank Spirit for guidance. Appreciating guidance opens you up to receive more!

Remember that if you are not calm, you are not likely to get a clear answer. That is one reason that the calming breath in the beginning of this exercise is so important. Remember also not to become dependent on using a pendulum for your decision making. Learn to center yourself, calm yourself, and ask Spirit for help. Trust that when you "ask, it shall be given to you."

PRACTICING INTUITIVE REIKI

During the afternoon I offer the students a traditional Japanese attunement, a *rei-ju*. This simple, beautiful ritual enhances the Reiki energy that flows through their hands and enhances their intuition even further.

Before we go to the bodywork tables to practice receiving impressions as we do hands-on Reiki, I review the symbols. I acknowledge that there are a variety of ways to draw and use the symbols. I also admit that there is a point at which the need for the symbols falls away in distant healing. The practitioner just raises his hands and the Reiki energy is already on its way to the client—and it is strong! However, my experience has taught me that each of the symbols focus the Reiki energy in a special way, rather like a prism refracts light. In addition to the commonly recognized purposes, the first symbol establishes protection; the second facilitates intuitive communication with the client and guidance; the third establishes sacred space and time and subtly alters the present moment to be more in harmony with Spirit. These qualities associated with each symbol may not be immediately apparent, but they reveal to us more aspects of the Reiki energy.

THE FIRST SYMBOL

While all advanced Reiki practitioners are aware of the first symbol as "the power symbol," which calls for an increase in Reiki energy over a particular area, not all are aware that this symbol is also immensely protective. The only way that I know to demonstrate this is to share stories of using the first symbol during a blizzard—and during a stroke.

Here is one story that I like to tell.

Several years ago, there was a blizzard that dropped thirty-six inches of snow on Philadelphia over the course of twenty-four hours. On that particular day I had an appointment, scheduled months in advance, with an accountant to go over my taxes, and no local weather forecaster warning of a severe storm system and hazardous road conditions was going to stop me. By 6 AM I was busy gathering up all the documents that I would need to show the accountant. By 7 AM I was on the road in my tiny hatchback car. The snowflakes were already falling thick and fast, adhering to the deep ruts of snow that covered the long driveway. By the time I got to the end of the driveway I was gripping the steering wheel with one hand and drawing the first symbol with the other, chanting its name over and over again.

I turned onto the unplowed country road and kept drawing and chanting, drawing and chanting. I drove very slowly and carefully. The trip to the nearest highway, which usually took ten minutes, took twenty-five minutes. As I turned onto this four-lane highway, which had been plowed and salted hours earlier, I realized that the blizzard was worsening. The snow was coating the road, and it was slick. I continued to drive slowly, drawing the first symbol, chanting its name. I could feel the Reiki energy buzzing all around me, and eventually I realized that I could see an area that I recognized as "safe passage" superimposed over the highway. It extended out from my car, about five feet on each side, and ahead of my car another couple of hundred feet. I knew that as long as I kept chanting the symbol and stayed within that area, I would be safe. And I was. Even though there were countless other cars in both lanes fish-tailing and swerving and ending up in snowbanks, I was safe.

When I arrived in Philadelphia I didn't look for a parking space on the street but headed right into a parking garage. Then I raced to keep my appointment. The accountant was ready to see, able to help me fill out my tax forms in under an hour, and surprised me with the good news that I would be getting a refund. I thanked the accountant and found my way down to street level again, where the snow quickly covered my coat. I decided that I wouldn't attempt the drive home yet and decided to drop in on a friend who lived nearby.

She was home, glad to make me a cup of tea and catch up on news. After a while we turned on the radio and listened to the announcements of airports and roads being closed in Philadelphia and New York. "You know, you aren't going to be able to drive home in this today," my friend said. "Why don't you just plan on staying the night on my couch?"

"Thank you," I said. "That sounds like a great idea." The day that followed was magical. We visited with my friend's downstairs neighbor, a photographer who was assembling his portfolio, and looked at his wonderful photos all afternoon. We watched people cross-country skiing down Spruce Street, now closed to traffic. We went out for dinner to a Chinese restaurant that stayed open because the cooks, the waiters, and waitresses all lived out of town, and they were snowed in too. We ended our snow day with a dart match at the local bar and a midnight visit to a rare bookstore to look at autographed first editions and rare folios—a thrill for a would-be writer.

Years later I still think of this snow day as one of the best days in my life because it unfolded like a flower, becoming more of a delight as each hour passed. I know that the Reiki energy, focused through the first symbol, protected me from harm on the road, but I've come to believe that it also moved ahead of me through time, making the day one of blessing after blessing.

Then I share another story. One of my Reiki students, who has had diabetes for many years, remembered the first symbol while she was having a stroke. As she felt herself losing consciousness, she visualized the symbol and chanted its name in her mind. When she woke up, she was in the hospital connected to monitors. After some testing the doctors were able to tell her that the damage to her brain was so minimal that it had already healed. She could go on about her life as before, with just a few simple lifestyle changes and with more awareness.

I encourage the students to remember the symbol's protective qualities, especially when they travel, wherever they go, and to use the symbol to begin the day with the brief meditation that follows. This meditation was taught to me by Tom Rigler, one of those responsible for bringing Japanese Reiki Master Hiroshi Doi and his knowledge of Japanese Reiki history and techniques to the West. This meditation is very easy to do and only takes a moment.

Meditation on the Symbols

This technique enables the practitioner to cultivate an awareness of the energetic qualities of each of the Reiki symbols. While it is recommended to begin practicing this meditation with the first symbol, the technique may be used with the other symbols as a way to become more conscious of the individual focus of Reiki energy that each one provides.

1. Standing in a relaxed posture, gassho.
2. Perform Kenyoko-ho.
3. Connect to Reiki light.
4. Gassho again, setting your intention to become more aware of the energy of the first Reiki symbol.
5. With your power hand, draw the first symbol, large, in front of you, an arm's-length away (fig. 14.2). Say or chant the sacred name of the symbol, as you have been taught.
6. Step forward into the energy of the symbol (fig. 14.3). Close your eyes for a moment (fig. 14.4). Feel the Reiki energy focused through the symbol transforming you.
7. Gassho. Be thankful for this experience.
8. Open your eyes and go about your day.

This meditation may be repeated with the same symbol to deepen your awareness of its distinct nature, or it may be done with each of the remaining Reiki symbols, in turn.

An alternate way to perform this meditation is as follows.

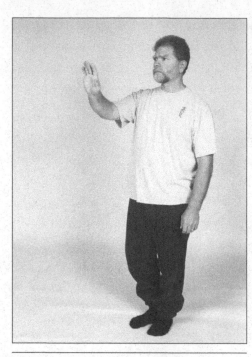

Figure 14.2

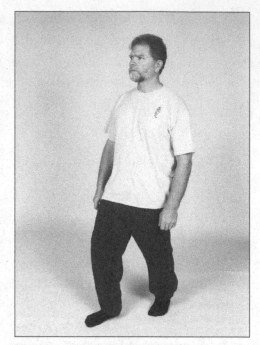

Figure 14.3

1. Sitting or standing in a relaxed, comfortable posture, gassho.
2. Perform Kenyoko-ho.
3. Connect to Reiki light.
4. Gassho again, setting your intention to become more aware of the subtle energy of the first Reiki symbol.
5. With your power hand, draw the first symbol, large, in front of you, an arm's-length away (fig. 14.5). Say or chant the sacred name of the symbol, as you have been taught.
6. With your physical hands, reach

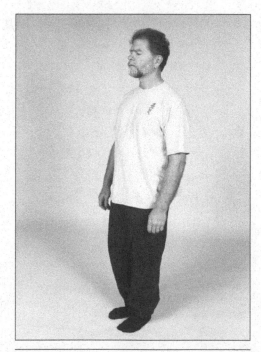

Figure 14.4

out and pick up the symbol, as if it were a piece of clothing you were removing from clips on a hanger (fig. 14.6). Clasp the symbol at its right and left edges with your fingertips and then bring your hands back to your shoulders, open your fingers, and drop the symbol down, over your shoulders, onto you (fig. 14.7). Close your eyes for a moment so that you can focus on the feeling of the Reiki energy embodied in that symbol now gently transforming you (fig. 14.8).

7. Gassho. Be thankful for this experience.
8. Open your eyes. Shake out your hands.

For the next half hour we work with only the first symbol, practicing its use for protection and increased Reiki energy. Then we review the second symbol, the mental-emotional healing symbol, and discuss how it can be used as the "talking symbol." Finally, we talk about the third symbol, the distant-healing symbol, and its ability to establish sacred time and space for the purpose of healing. Chanting this symbol can impact time in wonderful ways.

Then we practice at the bodywork table, receiving intuitive impressions, describing them to the client, listening to the client's comments. Sometimes the students receive only a few impressions that come in a flash or float slowly into the mind. Others are able to enjoy the exchange of information that comes through intuitive dialogue. Occasionally a student will have the experience of impressions coming so quickly that dialogue is not possible. The client is engaged in a monologue, and the student is privileged to listen and witness another's concerns and cares.

When all the students have had a chance to practice we return to our seats to do some distant healing, again with the awareness that it is possible to receive intuitive impressions that support Reiki healing. The afternoon ends with another Japanese-style attunement and instruction in listening to the sensations of energy in the hands (hibiki), scanning the body for areas in need of healing (Byosen-ho), and asking the Reiki energy to guide the course of the treatment (Reiji-ho). It is gratifying that the practitioners are quickly able to understand and to use these techniques.

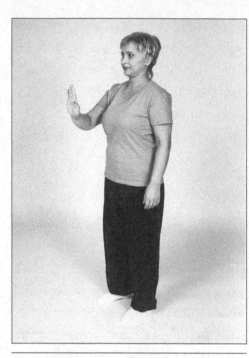

Figure 14.5

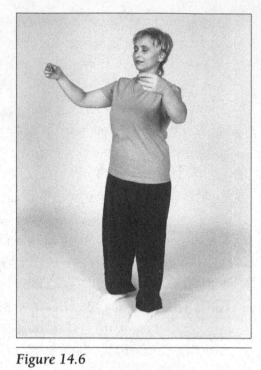

Figure 14.6

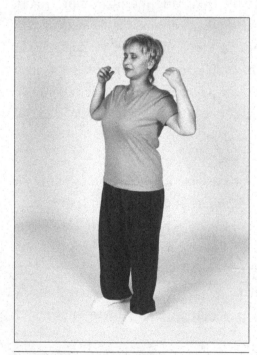

Figure 14.7

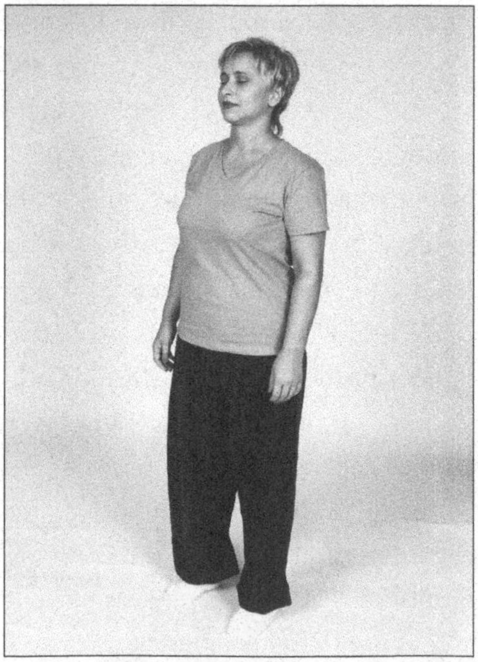

Figure 14.8

Meditations Using the First Symbol

1. Standing at ease, physically draw the first symbol in front of you and walk into its energy. Enjoy wearing the Reiki energy all day.

2. Standing at ease, physically draw the first symbol in front of you, pick it up as if it was a shirt on a line, and put it on by transferring it to yourself. Again, enjoy the added Reiki energy and protection.

3. As you stand, sit in a chair, or kneel or sit cross-legged on the floor, visualize a large first symbol coming in from above your head, slightly to your left, going straight down through the vertical center of your body into the earth, and spiraling up to finally touch your heart. This increases the Reiki energy flowing through you, centers and grounds you, and adds protection.

4. As you stand, sit in a chair, or kneel or sit cross-legged on the floor, visualize the first symbol, small in size (about 3 inches), floating in front of your heart and in back of you, at the level of your heart. This symbol is protective, increases Reiki energy, and helps you connect with others through unconditional love.

5. As you stand, sit in a chair, or kneel or sit cross-legged on the floor, visualize the first symbol, small in size (about 3 inches), at the back of each chakra, starting with the crown, then the third eye, the throat, the heart, the solar plexus, the spleen, the root. Then visualize the first symbol, large, extending from overhead down through your crown, along your spine, to under your feet, to ground you. This meditation is protective and centering and calls for an increase in Reiki energy.

6. While standing or sitting in a chair visualize a large horizontal first symbol entering you at your heart. Extend the spirals downward around your body, finally into the earth below. Visualize another large, horizontal first symbol entering you at your heart. Extend the spirals upward around your body, finally into heaven above. Follow this with another visualization of a large vertical first symbol extending through your center from overhead to under feet, to ground you. This technique cleanses and clears the chakras, centers and grounds you, and calls for an increase in Reiki energy.

7. Combine meditations on the first symbol as you feel guided. For example, visualize a large vertical first symbol through your body, then two smaller first symbols, one in front and one behind you, at the level of your heart. Enjoy the feeling of being aligned with Spirit, grounded and heart-centered in the Reiki energy.

   Repetition of the first symbol is allowed and encouraged. Three repetitions links the exercise with the "call to Spirit" that is associated with the call to prayer across culture and religions. (As always in Reiki, remember to say the name of the symbol three times whenever you physically draw or visualize it.)

On the second day of the Reiki and Intuition Workshop we explore territory that is entirely new to most of the practitioners: doing intuitive readings of a person, a photograph, an object, and drawing the aura or energy field. With the permission of intuitive reader, teacher, and Reiki Master Linda Schiller-Hanna, we try a step-by-step exercise she uses in her intuitive development classes, and then we practice it, adapted for use with the Reiki energy and symbols.

A Method for Working with Reiki to Receive Intuitive Guidance for a Partner

1. As you sit facing your client, breathe a relaxing, centering breath of Reiki as light, imagining you can inhale through the top of your head and fill up not only your lungs but your whole body, all the way down to your feet and even below your feet. Breathe in to relax, calm, ground, and center yourself. Breathe in to invite Spirit to fill your energy body with light. Reiki practitioners who feel guided to do so may use the first symbol while doing an intuitive reading for a client to call for additional protection and healing from the energy (fig. 14.9).

2. Perform Kenyoko-ho, Dry Brushing, to clear your energy field. Then raise your arms up high, Reiki hands on and open, and slowly lower your arms, sending Reiki into your energy field and physical body to heal you of any sense of discomfort, tension, or stress. As you "shower" you may visualize

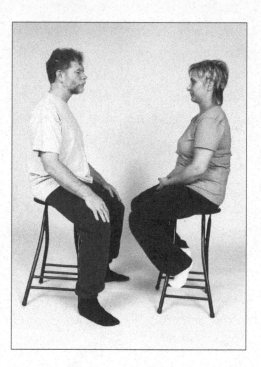

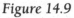

Figure 14.9

Reiki as beautiful sparkling drops of light gently raining down on you and clearing away any negativity, disharmony, discord, or distress. Support this visualization with your intention.

3. Again raise your arms up high, Reiki hands on and open, and ask for the light of Reiki to come down over you as you lower your hands into gassho, or prayer position, so that you now stand or sit within a column of white light. As you continue with the reading, maintain a relaxed awareness that you are within this column, breathing in the light of Reiki and radiating the light of Reiki.

4. Pray to Spirit in whatever way feels most appropriate to you, asking for divine protection and guidance for yourself and your client. Set your intention to be accurate, truthful, clear, and kind in relaying any impressions you receive, so that you may serve the highest good.

5. Relax. Continue to breathe in the light of Reiki and radiate the light of Reiki. If you notice any areas of physical stress or tension that remain in your body, ask the Reiki energy to go there so that you can be more comfortable as you do the reading.

6. With your eyes open, make a heart connection with your client. Visualize an arc or rainbow cord of light that extends from your own heart to that of the client.

7. Close your eyes, extend your Reiki hands toward your client, and ask your client (whose eyes should remain open) to say his or her name three times.

8. Allow yourself to notice whatever impressions come and describe them to your client as they occur, without waiting for any client response. Continue for as long as the impressions come. If the client asks for clarification or makes a comment during the reading, let yourself be gently redirected to notice whatever impressions come in response. Feel free to move your hands around, up and down, side to side, as you sense the client's energy field (fig. 14.10).

9. When you feel intuitively that you are finished or no more impressions come, let the client know the reading is over, open your eyes, and be willing to review your impressions with the client while they are still fresh in your mind (fig. 14.11). Be gentle, tactful, and remember, "just for today, be kind."

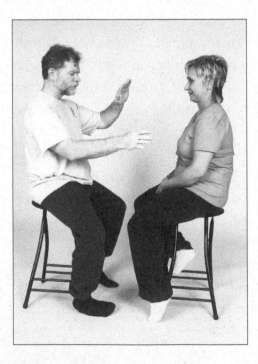

Figure 14.10

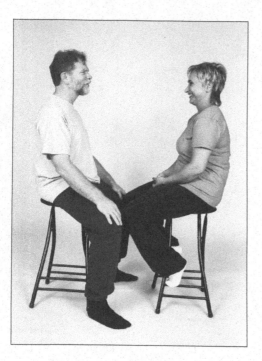

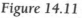

Figure 14.11

10. Visualize the arc or rainbow cord of light connecting your hearts now dissolving, breaking, being cut, or withdrawing. Thank your client and give thanks to Spirit for allowing you to act as a channel for healing and guidance in another way.

With practice, the ritualized techniques of Kenyoko-ho and Reiki shower may simply be visualized. However, extending Reiki hands into the client's energy field seems to be essential to the success of the reading, as it allows the practitioner to listen to subtle changes and notice what Reiki brings to conscious awareness as impressions.

Reiki practitioners who practice these techniques are often surprised to discover how easy they become with repetition. When the practitioner feels the client's energy field with Reiki-charged hands, intuitive impressions arise naturally on the flow of subtle energy. Even practitioners who claim that they have never seen an aura discover that, immersed in the Reiki energy, they can "know" what color crayons to choose to draw their impressions of the client's energy field (fig. 14.12). They can sense something about the unknown owner of a set of keys or

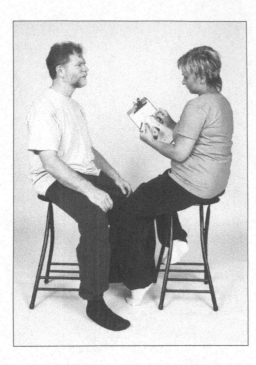

Figure 14.12

a watch or a pet's collar. They can even become aware of possible past lives that may be impacting the client's life today.

Any Reiki practitioner who has been trained in traditional intuitive Reiki techniques and developed a foundation of experience can sense information about the client's energy field, and about relationships and events, even in the very distant past, that are affecting the client's health and well-being now. The above methods are offered to practitioners not to replace any Reiki techniques, but to help the practitioner more quickly develop confidence and become comfortable presenting intuitive impressions to the client.

SUGGESTIONS FOR PRACTITIONERS

While reading a book cannot give you the same depth of experience as attending a class and practicing what is taught, this chapter provides a fair sampling of the techniques that are presented at a Reiki and Intuition Workshop. Experiment with whatever exercises feel right to you. This is an opportunity to go deeper into your practice of Reiki, to become more comfortable with the symbols, and to explore how Reiki supports intuition at the bodywork table, during distant healing, and in "ordinary" life. The invitation is straightforward: to become more aware of Reiki as a conscious connection to Spirit and of intuition as the voice of the soul.

NOW YOU

While you might begin your exploration of these techniques anywhere that feels appropriate, becoming more conscious of the protective qualities of the first symbol is an excellent place to start. Call on the Reiki energy to increase the healing around you and to protect you by using the first symbol wherever you can in your daily life: as you rise to face the day, at the steering wheel of your car, as you enter your workplace, as you prepare to eat a meal, as you wave good-bye to a friend, as you turn down the covers of your bed at night. Allow the Reiki energy, through your use of the first symbol, to gently transform your world into a safer, healthier place.

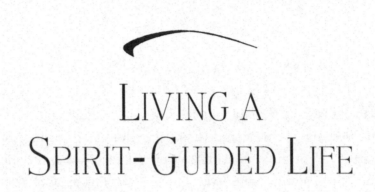

LIVING A
SPIRIT-GUIDED LIFE

When we allow ourselves to be guided by Spirit, we begin to live again in a state of grace. We give conscious, willing attention to Spirit, ask for guidance, and receive, in return, the sense that each day brings countless blessings. When we first begin to practice Reiki most of us do not consciously know that this can occur—and will occur, if we practice with commitment. Yet the experiences we have in Reiki are so fulfilling, so fascinating, that most practitioners feel compelled to do more: we join a Reikishare; we take groceries and good cheer to a housebound elderly neighbor once a week, hoping for a chance to offer Reiki; we give Reiki to runners at the finish line of a race; we volunteer at a hospital or hospice; we help in a soup kitchen on Thanksgiving, feeling our hands radiating healing into every scoop of filling we dish out.

Our commitment brings many rewards, the simplest of these being the knowledge that we are living our lives from a place of compassion; we are acting with integrity; we are doing what is right. This satisfies heart, mind, soul. Our self-respect heals and our self-esteem improves. As we become able to acknowledge the Source of our own healing, it occurs to us that we can ask for even more. We enter into a conversation with Spirit that may begin in meditation or prayer or Reiki self-treatment at the start of the day. We feel the flow of unconditional love. We feel gratitude. We say, "Please help me with this, God," or "Thank you, Spirit"—and the conversation never stops. As we "listen" to the energy of Spirit we enjoy companionship, love, laughter, awe, reverence, gratitude, grace.

This does not happen overnight. We learn Reiki, not knowing on a conscious level that we now have a much stronger, clearer connection to Spirit. We practice Reiki and through practice, over time, recognize this connection to Spirit and realize its nature. We commit to practice, now conscious of this connection, asking Spirit to guide us in our client work and in our lives. We open to receive whatever opportunities for service Spirit brings our way. Tentatively, we begin to live our lives in conversation with Spirit. We ask to be guided to those opportunities. We ask for help as we offer healing. We receive guidance and help, but we don't always recognize it. Yet as we remain committed to Reiki and to our spiritual path, as we continue to ask, we do begin to recognize, appreciate, and honor the guidance we receive.

AN EARLY LESSON IN INTENTION

About six weeks after my advanced Reiki training in 1987, my boyfriend and I were driving south on Route 95 through the Old City section of Philadelphia. The October sky was bright blue, the sunlight dazzling, the air crisp and cool—a perfect day. I sat in the passenger seat beside him, my hands relaxed in my lap, my attention on our conversation.

Suddenly my hands began to radiate Reiki energy and heat up like stadium lights. I raised them up, looking at them in awe, and looked around to see what might be calling for the energy. Nothing. We were still heading south on 95, with few cars around us, just entering the high, concrete-walled curve near the Washington Avenue exit. My hands pulsed with heat. I looked at them in confusion, not understanding. The cars ahead of us began to slow. Within about fifteen seconds they stopped, and we slowed to a stop as well.

All I could think was that there must have been an accident on the road ahead of us, around the curve, beyond my line of sight. My hands, which I still held up in the air, fingers spread, were radiating Reiki with an intensity that I had never before experienced. Someone in that accident needed healing. What was I supposed to do?

I had no medical training, not even current Red Cross first aid or CPR certification. I had no "legitimate" excuse to get out of the car, walk to the scene of the accident, and offer my help. So I sat in the car, frozen with confusion, my hands raised, radiating Reiki energy to people I could not see, had never met, would never meet. I didn't know whether to feel appalled by my cowardice or awed by the power of Reiki—or both.

We waited in the car for about forty-five minutes while policemen and rescue workers saw to the people involved in the accident, and tow trucks cleared the wreckage. That evening, on the television news, I saw still photos of the multi-vehicle collision for the first time. I looked again at my hands, hoping that some of the Reiki energy they had radiated so intensely had actually been received by those in need.

When I next assisted at a Reiki class with Beth Gray, I asked her about my experience. "What should I have done? What *could* I have done?" I wanted to know. She told me that all I needed to do was raise my hands up, palms facing in the direction of the accident. The Reiki energy would go to those in need.

I thought about what I had done, simply raising my hands up to look at them, and holding them up, my fingers spread, as they radiated heat and pulsing the air. At least I had been guided to do that much. Was that enough? Was it any help at all to those people who were involved in the accident? I hoped so. I prayed so.

Years later, when I first began to teach Reiki, some of my students challenged me about the nature of intention. "Intention is everything," they said. *No*, I thought, *divine intention is everything*. Reiki practitioners can commit to service, align ourselves with the flow of energy, ask for guidance, and release the outcome. Spirit intends and accomplishes the work of healing.

Many years have passed since this experience with the Reiki energy, but I still find it a great comfort to know that Spirit can use me as a channel whether I am ready, prepared, focused, and attentive—or not. I am grateful that my faults and imperfections do not impede the flow of Reiki energy or Spirit's healing by so much as a single atom or wave/particle of light.

THE LESSON IS LOVE

As we continue to engage in conversation with Spirit, asking for more opportunities to be of service and to offer healing, we are often guided by an inner impulse to do something out of the ordinary, to set aside doubts for the moment to see what Spirit wants to bring our way. Here are two stories about being guided to find right work.

Barbara Sautter, a Reiki Master who felt secure in her position as office manager in her brother's business, felt perplexed when he sold his company and she found herself suddenly unemployed. Reminded to follow her guidance by sitting in on a Reiki and Intuition Workshop, she began job hunting. On her way from an interview with an employment agency she found herself stopping at an intersection that she had planned to drive through, turning down a side street, and stopping the car in front of a chiropractor's office that she had never seen before. Still following her inner guidance, she walked up the steps to the office, went in, and introduced herself. Because someone on the staff was leaving, the chiropractor anticipated a need for someone with her skills within a short time. Would she please leave her resume?

Connie Seneko, an unemployed nurse, decided she would volunteer to do Reiki at a local hospice while she waited for the right position to come along. When a job fair was advertised in her neighborhood, she called me and told me that she felt guided to go to this fair. She had a good feeling about it. My own guidance, as I spoke with her on the phone, tallied with hers. I encouraged her to be confident, optimistic, and let her light shine as she smiled and shook hands and talked with potential employers. At the job fair she spoke to a fellow nursing professional whom she immediately liked and respected. This woman invited her to an interview and hired her within the month to work in a position she loves.

As we continue to work with Reiki, consciously aligning our will with that of

Spirit to support healing that is for the highest good, we are sometimes guided to use a level of intention or additional healing modalities. Here, a Reiki Master who works as an ecologist for the park service describes using intuitive Reiki in a directive way to help save a bat colony.

> I use Reiki to connect with wild animals so they lose their fear and I can "talk" with them. As the bat expert, I get a lot of frantic calls during the summer. Reiki prayers are a big part of this work. One summer a bat tested positive for rabies and the health department overreacted by ordering the extermination of the entire colony (which past research has shown is not at all necessary). My bosses left me no choice but to allow the activity and I felt terrible and helpless about it, until I thought about Reiki. I sent Reiki to the situation for everyone's highest good, but I also tried to connect with the colony. I told them they had to leave or they would get killed, and I told them to take their babies too. I called the next day to find out about the travesty and was told that there were no bats—over one hundred bats had just vanished and were nowhere to be found! No one was more surprised than I was.

The story that follows describes how another Reiki Master was guided to use Reiki with creative visualization to support her client's healing. Noreen Ryen, a massage therapist, had been traveling around the United States and Canada in a caravan for almost a year, when her route took her into the Southwest. She wrote the following from Mesa Verde.

> We visited a few of the Pueblo ruins yesterday. Our Park Ranger guide approached her presentation on a spiritual note, describing the Native Americans and their ceremonies with great respect. I knew from the start this was a special gift. I was overcome with emotion.
>
> At tour's end I thanked the ranger. I felt driven to hug her and then went on my way. Later that day, didn't I bump into her again at another site? This time she shared more with me. She started to tell me about the Native American belief in People of Light, then stopped midsentence to say she had goose bumps all over her body. She trusted her body was helping

her recognize something of the light in me. It was then that I told her about Reiki. She said that she felt I had been meant to return to this place. She said I might now begin to see signs in my meditations—signs that would help me in my journey.

Finally, she told me of a chronic pain she has in her forearm. I asked permission to lay my hands on the area and immediately felt her bones grinding together. I had an intuitive sense that she had broken her wrist in an earlier existence. I shared this impression with her. I felt guided to visualize the bones of her wrist coming together and completely healing as I gave her Reiki. As we stood by the ruins her arm bones moved under my hands, then the muscles relaxed, and she said she felt better. As she was on duty, this happened in just a few minutes, and I was sorry we wouldn't meet again.

FEEL THE LOVE AND LET GO

As we become more comfortable listening to the Reiki energy in our hands and listening to Spirit, accepting Spirit's guidance, it occurs to us to ask for approval of our intentions and our choices. Sometimes this means that we offer a client silent, soul-level encouragement to take a particular course of action, if it is for the highest good. Sometimes this means that we honor the guidance we receive by adding another holistic healing method to the Reiki we are already using. Sometimes this means we accept that all our best efforts will not change an outcome. We surrender to Spirit and discover that we are supported in accepting loss.

When I was a child my parents would often tell stories or sing to my brother and me when we took a long car ride. Since all of our relatives lived at least an hour's drive away, we shared some wonderful stories and sang many songs. One of my favorites was an American folk song called "Frog Went A-Courting." My father would sing Frog's proposal to my mother: "Miss Mousie, would you marry me?" and my mother, a.k.a. Miss Mousie, would sing in reply: "Uh-uh." (That's a "yes" in mouse language, in case you can't tell.) Watching and listening to my parents sing this song to each other, I knew, even at six years old, that their love for one another would last a lifetime.

Sadly, a lifetime passes too quickly. In the late 1990s my mother began to suffer from a debilitating illness that was never successfully diagnosed, though doctors at several hospitals tested her for many different conditions. In 2000 my father and I became her caretakers for the last four years of her life, during which time she grew weaker and was more and more often confined to her bed. We fed her, though there was little that she could eat. I used Reiki to help her swallow and to ease the pain and numbness of neuropathy in her feet and legs. To keep my mother's spirits up I made sure she was well stocked with books by her favorite authors, and I often sat with her and talked, just to keep her company.

During the summer of 2003 her condition worsened. During the fall, one of the visiting nurses who came twice a week to check my mother's dressings and check her vital signs recommended that we think about hospice care. She didn't expect my mother to live more than a few months.

Knowing that the Thanksgiving that approached would probably be my mother's last, we talked with the rest of my family about what we could do to make it special. I remembered that earlier in the year I had taught Reiki I to a professional harpist, who was also a lay minister. I called her and asked if there was any way that she could come make time in her busy schedule for a home visit.

The harpist was kind enough to come in the early afternoon of the day before Thanksgiving. Although we were a very small audience, we were an appreciative one. She played many of my mother's favorite songs and hymns, including "Lord of the Dance" and "Ave Maria." My mother looked on, smiling in wonder, like a small child. Finally, after we were all feeling transformed by the echoing notes and chords of joyful sound and song, the harpist put away her harp and asked if she might pray with my mother, who willingly accepted. Here was an unasked-for kindness, a blessing that touched all our hearts.

We thanked the harpist again and again, wished her a happy Thanksgiving, and watched out the window as she drove away. Then my father helped my mother back to bed, my aunt and my mother's best friend went home, and my sister-in-law and I drove to the grocery store. Although we had several items to pick up, we made our way directly to the special display where the turkeys were stocked to pick out a bird.

We looked down into a cavernous hold. There were a couple of capons, a goose, a few ducks—but no turkeys. We debated what to do. My sister-in-law suggested that a ham might do. I said no, I thought we really should do our best to find a turkey. I had promised to feed seven people Thanksgiving dinner the next day, one of whom was not likely to be with us the next time this holiday came round. We had to have a turkey. I wandered over to the dairy case, chewing my lip, thinking about what to do next. I turned to my sister-in-law. "Maybe if we go to another grocery store . . . ?"

Suddenly I noticed a clerk toweling off his hands near us. I walked up to him and asked him if there were any more turkeys in the back. "No, that's it," he said. "They were gone earlier this afternoon."

"Thanks," I said and drifted back to stand by my sister-in-law, who was still staring down into the empty case.

"Say, are you two together?" the clerk asked.

We nodded.

"Were you planning to have Thanksgiving together?"

We nodded again.

"Well, maybe I can help you out then," the clerk began. "My wife just called to tell me that we're not having Thanksgiving at home. We got invited to spend it with some folks from the firehouse, and she wants to do that. So I have a twenty-two-pound turkey in the back that's already started thawing out. You can have that if you want it."

My sister-in-law's eyes shimmered with tears. "That we would be wonderful," I said. "Thank you. You're very kind to help us."

The clerk looked down, almost shyly. "Well, I'll just step in the back and get it then." He turned, pushed open one of the white double doors into the warehouse, and disappeared into the darkness.

"This kind of thing never happens in real life," my sister-in-law said in astonishment.

"Then consider it a miracle that arrived just when we needed one," I told her. "Now we have something more to be grateful about tomorrow."

"He doesn't even realize . . ."

"No," I said, "he has no idea how important his action is—and we don't have to tell him."

Just then the clerk emerged from the warehouse with an enormous turkey in its plastic wrapper held in his arms. He brought it over to us and set it down in the grocery cart. "Well, that's it," he said.

"Thank you," we said. "We'll say a special prayer for you tomorrow. Thank you so much."

The next day, because of this man's kindness, we were able to gather around a traditional Thanksgiving table as a family. My mother, in her robe, sat at one end, looking tiny and frail but very happy. My father sat at the other end, pleased to be surrounded by family. We all felt grateful to be together and to be able to celebrate the many blessings—expected and unexpected—of this holiday.

Early one evening a week later, my mother had a seizure. My father called 911, and an ambulance arrived within a couple of minutes, despite a raging snowstorm. Paramedics took my mother to the hospital's emergency room, where she was treated and then moved to a regular hospital room for observation. Because of the blizzard conditions, we did not follow the ambulance.

Instead, around eleven o'clock that night, when the snowstorm had finally subsided, my father looked out the front window into the darkness and noticed the deer. He called for me and we watched as a herd of deer crossed the snow-covered road from the cornfield into the front yard, then walked around the side of the house to the back. They scrabbled for seeds under the bird feeder, and then they settled down to stay for the night under the huge sheltering branches of a giant pine. There were ten of them, a buck, does, fawns. Even in the darkness we could see their silhouettes.

After my father went to bed, I continued to sit in the darkness and look out my bedroom window, so that I could watch the deer. Intuitively I knew they were guardians, watchers in the dark, and messengers, ten in all. I knew that whatever happened to my mother, their presence in some way marked a new beginning. (Numerologists associate the number ten with a new beginning.) I also connected them to Reiki, because, for me, deer have so often signified the presence of Spirit that I experience in Reiki. I knew that they brought healing for my mother and for my family. Several times when I woke from my anxious sleep that night I looked out the window again for them, and they were still there.

The next morning they were gone (although they returned night after night through the weeks that followed). I woke before my father and went to the living room to raise the blinds on the new day. The sky was white with the threat of more snow, and the snow that had fallen during the blizzard lay on the ground in deep white drifts that covered the porch and swept right up against the front door. Only the blue shadows of the tracks of the deer marked it.

Suddenly, an unfamiliar Jeep with a plow attached to the front of it backed into our driveway. The unknown driver backed up all the way to the garage, lowered the plow, pushed a single wide swath of snow out of the way, and drove off without a hello or good-bye. I said a silent thank you to the driver and to Spirit. This unasked-for kindness meant that we would be able to get to the hospital right away. When my father and I discussed this later he told me that he thought someone from the ambulance crew must have driven the Jeep and done the plowing. To me, knowing who the driver was makes no difference. The kindness, so unexpected and so powerful, was another sign that we were not alone. We were supported and surrounded and sheltered by love, both human and divine. Everything was being guided by Spirit.

My mother was admitted into the hospital on December 5th, 2003, with pneumonia and a blood infection. During the next four weeks she was in and out of coma, on and off of life support. She underwent difficult surgeries she was not expect to survive, and finally, we were told, would soon be able to come home.

On January 5th, my mother was moved to a regular hospital room. That day I looked up telephone numbers and addresses of rehabilitation facilities that had been recommended to us, and began to make inquires. That evening, thinking that my mother was soon going to be released from the hospital, I debated driving down to visit. I felt so tired. I had visited her every day, sometimes two or three times in a day, since she had been admitted. I had spent almost all of New Year's Eve at her bedside, from a little after dawn to a few minutes before midnight. Soon she would be coming home. Surely, I could, in good conscience, miss one night's visit.

Because I felt so bleary and befuddled, I used my pendulum to ask for guidance: "Mother-Father God, would you please guide the pendulum?" I saw the familiar back-and-forth motion.

"Will you please show me 'yes'?" Again, I saw the back-and-forth motion.

"Will you please show me 'no'?" The side-to-side swing that I expected followed.

"Is it for the highest good for me to take a night off from visiting my mother in the hospital?"

The pendulum swung side to side in a strong, wide arc.

I felt surprised—and frustrated. I was so weary. I wanted so much to have an early evening and a good night's rest. So I asked the question again, another way, and then again. No matter how I asked the question I received the same guidance: go to the hospital. So, with winter's early sunset already fading from the sky, I drove the distance.

My mother was alone. I pulled up a chair to sit with her and hold her hand and give her Reiki. She smiled at me in greeting. She seemed to have difficulty talking, but this did not surprise me, as she had some incisions on the sides of her throat that were still healing. She seemed to be looking beyond me. She put her hands together, as if to pray.

"Do you want me to pray with you?" I asked her.

She nodded, and I prayed with her. Because it was late, and the nurses were hovering near to turn down her lights for the night, I stayed only a few minutes more.

"I love you," I told her. She smiled and started to tell me the same. I stopped her. "No, save your voice," I told her. "I know you love me. I'll see you tomorrow. Sleep well." I kissed her good night, she settled back against the pillows, and I left the room.

Driving home in the darkness, I thought about how my mother had asked me to pray with her, and about how that had comforted her. I was glad that I had listened to the guidance I had received and made this visit.

The next day I had lunch with a Reiki Master friend. Confident that my mother was coming home soon, I relaxed for the first time in weeks. I was happy for my friend because he had just started to teach Reiki. I drove from the restaurant to the hospital, feeling better.

A doctor met me in the hallway outside my mother's room, a grim expression on her face. "Your mother is dying," she said. "We have her on morphine. There is nothing more that we can do." Stunned, I went into the room to be with her and to give her Reiki as she died. It was time to let her go.

The days until my mother's funeral passed in a blur. The service, in a beautiful country church that she had loved, felt like a celebration. The eulogy reminded the mourners of one of my mother's favorite quotations from the Bible: "This is the day the Lord hath made. Rejoice and be glad in it." The harpist's music lifted everyone's spirits. Family and friends remembered her with kindness and love, comforting one another.

The day after my mother's funeral, I wrote thank you notes to everyone who had attended or helped in any way. I knew that if I didn't immediately face the task, my grief would make me avoid it. Riding on the euphoria of the day before and supported by Reiki energy, which I knew many friends were still sending, I wrote from about nine in the morning to four in the afternoon. Finally, as I finished the last note, I felt my own grief overwhelming me, and I cried.

The next morning I woke earlier than anyone else in the house. I looked out the bay window in the living room at another brilliantly cold January day. I saw its bleakness and I felt the vastness of my sense of loss—and then, as I looked down, I noticed something moving in the leaves at the edge of the porch. I could not make out what was causing the motion, but I watched it move back and forth, just under the leaves, lifting them up and separating them like the crack of an earthquake, again and again. What could it be? I wondered. What creature would move like that on a January day when the temperature was not even 10 degrees Fahrenheit? The motion under the leaves extended for perhaps fifteen feet—back and forth, back and forth. I decided to watch the front edge of the movement to see if I might catch a glimpse of this creature. On about the twentieth circuit, a few of the leaves tipped away just enough to reveal a bit of gray-brown fur. A field mouse? As soon as I guessed the identity of my visitor, she completed the last circuit, hopped into a small terra cotta flower pot laying on its side, stood up, and looked right at me. She studied me over her shoulder for a long moment, and then scurried away, as if to say, "Well, you might have all day to stare out the window, but I have things to do!" I burst out laughing.

And I understood something: my mother, who had sung the part of Miss Mousie so many years ago and who had described herself all her life as having "mousy-brown hair," had arranged this morning's comedy for me. She didn't want me to fall into depression and sadness in the aftermath of her death. She wanted me to remember the happy times—and to know that, where she is, all is well. I set aside my sadness in that moment. I knew that I would feel sad again, but I also understood that I was not to make grief my focus, as I had made caretaking. I was to come back to life and to reconnect to my work in this world. Thanks to the visit of a little mouse, I understood that I would do so with her blessing.

RETURNED TO LIFE

Glenda Johnson, a Reiki Master from Kansas City, shared her story with me as we sat in the lobby of the Grand Hotel in Toronto the day before the Usui Reiki Ryoho Conference in October 2002. Ten years ago, she told me, she had cancer. In 1989, about three weeks after she learned Reiki, physicians did an MRI and made the diagnosis. They found several tumors in her abdomen and wanted to schedule surgery as soon as possible.

"Did you use Reiki to treat yourself?" I asked her.

"When the pain started," she explained, "I was already in what the doctors called 'the last stage.' It hurt so badly that I couldn't stop myself from screaming. My hands would turn into claws. Every muscle in my body would become rigid. It was pretty bad. The only thing that stopped the pain or that eased the pain was to do Reiki."

"Did you have any support?"

"I called my friend who had brought me to Reiki and asked her to contact the others who were in our class. They were all friends of hers. I requested that she contact our Reiki Master, and the Reiki Master put my name into the Reiki circle the next day. She called and told me that everyone in the Reiki circle—all of the Reiki people she knew—were going to be sending me long-distance healing. So I wasn't the only one doing all the Reiki."

"Did you still have the operation?"

"Yes, I did, but a week before the operation, in the middle of the night, I had a near-death experience. I had one of those attacks of pain, and I was giving myself Reiki. It was all I could do to move my hands from one position to the next.

"Then my bedroom started lighting up with this golden light. I *was* awake —this was not a waking dream. I looked in the corner of my room and saw this intense golden light, with white light pulsing through it. With every pulse more light filled the room, until there were no shadows. It was as if the light was going through everything.

"And the light became an angel, and the angel said that he had come for me, and I said to him, 'No, I'm not feeling easy about this.' And he said to me, 'I'm going to show you your life experience.'

"He did a life review with me, and he explained why I had met everyone in my life and what our contract had been. I had fulfilled the mission that I had contracted for in this lifetime, and I was ready to go.

"Then he showed me where I was going to be going. It was just beautiful. There were flowers and parkways, and in the distance there was this beautiful city, and it was white with green spires and domes—a lot like Puttaparthi in India, actually, where Sai Baba has a great center of learning. And the angel said, 'You can go with me now to this place.'

"And I said, 'Well, I just became a Reiki channel, and if it is true that I have fulfilled my mission, I would like to stay and help others with theirs.' I asked if he knew what Reiki was, and he laughed, and I heard bells sounding. It was just beautiful. I can't describe it.

"And he explained that Reiki was the healing power of the universe brought closer to the earth in the laying on of hands, that it was a true healing spirit.

"When we were done talking the light started going back into him, and he disappeared with a pop," she said, clapping her hands once, "like that! He was gone.

"When they opened me up on the operating table a week later, the pathologist was standing by. He looked into my open body, and he said, 'That's cancer.'

He turned around and walked out. It was that bad. The other doctor was just going to close me up, but he had this thought come into his head: 'Let's wait a minute before we close her up.' . . . He sent a frozen section down to the lab; the same pathologist that had seen me opened up a few minutes before was now in the lab. He said, 'This can't be. Are you sure this is from that patient? There are *no* cancer cells.' So they removed the noncancerous tumors, and they removed the parts of me that were ruined by the noncancerous tumors, and they sewed me up—and I never went through chemotherapy or radiation."

Glenda closed her story with a shy smile, clearly at peace with herself and her new life purpose. I thanked her, and thanked Spirit for bringing me to this place, to this person, to this moment in time, to hear her story.

Harmony. Grace. Connection to Spirit. Whether we live through times of joy or times of sorrow, it is possible to feel the resonance of the energy permeating our days, guiding us step by step, moment by moment, sometimes breath by breath. It is possible, by being aware of inner guidance and by reading the "signs"—the synchronicities that are the outward evidence of guidance—to know that we are supported and infinitely loved. There is nothing more beautiful to a soul who has longed for a connection to Spirit than to know this comfort.

SUGGESTIONS FOR PRACTITIONERS

Reflect on your commitment to Reiki and how it has changed over time since you became a practitioner. Have you ever consciously deepened your commitment? Have you ever thought about how reevaluating your practice and looking for ways to renew your commitment might bring rewards?

Would it feel good to you to do some volunteer work with Reiki or to retrain at a particular level or recharge yourself by assisting at a class? All of these opportunities are available to you. Each of them can give you the chance to immerse yourself in the Reiki energy for a few hours or for a day and to heal in ways that are divinely intended just for you.

Those with many years of Reiki experience can still benefit from recognizing the value of consciously recommitting to practice. You know well the wild joy that witnessing unexpected healing brings. You also know the simple pleasure of feeling subtle, positive shifts in yourself each day, as you heal within, and you've recognized how your external life has changed to mirror that healing.

While there are annual Reiki retreats in some locations, which provide wonderful experiences of Reiki in community, going within and being fully present to your own experience of Reiki in the quiet of your own home for an hour or two can offer you a profound sense of healing and renewal. Take advantage of this opportunity often to go deeper, to discover purpose, to find guidance.

NOW YOU

Block out a chunk of uninterrupted time, perhaps a whole morning or an afternoon, where you can do Reiki on yourself. Unplug the phone or turn off the ringer. Turn off your cell phone, if you carry one. Go to a space that you consider sanctuary. This might be your bedroom, a meditation room, or a client treatment room, or it might be an outdoor space—a cliff-top view of a canyon, a grassy spot on a bank beside a stream, a clearing in the woods—a place where you can claim solitude.

Make yourself comfortable lying on your back. Treat yourself with Reiki. Listen to the energy in your hands. When your attention wanders from the energy, gently, lovingly, bring it back. Listen. Notice everything you feel: heat, coolness, current, pressure, tingles, prickles, whirls, pulses, waves. Keep listening. When you feel the shift in energy in your hands that would normally signal you to move your hands to another position, stay where you are. Listen to the energy as it slowly—or quickly—rises again, maybe quieter this time, maybe more intense. Listen to the dance of energy in your hands and feel the dance of atoms under your hands as your own body heals. Listen through another cycle of the energy, and another, and another—until your hands are completely quiet.

Then move your hands to the next position. Listen, with the same loving attention, to the sensations of energy in your hands again. Listen through cycle after cycle until, once more, your hands are completely quiet. Then move your hands to the next position. In this way, complete an entire treatment. Be willing to give yourself the time to experience the extraordinary sense of well-being, peace, and happiness that follows.

Know that you can give yourself this experience again, that you can use it to prepare yourself to treat a client, or to go into meditation, or to teach. Understand that you can ask to be guided, hand position by hand position, through this experience, or that you can follow the pattern of positions you were taught. Understand that doing Reiki on yourself this way is a kind of meditation itself. Ask to be guided, and whatever impressions come, be at peace in Spirit.

16

INTUITIVE REIKI IN SERVICE TO SPIRIT: CONVERSATIONS WITH REIKI MASTERS

Perhaps nothing can reinforce the value of intuition for spiritual pathwork so much as hearing well-known Reiki Masters share their own stories. Some of these individuals were clearly guided by intuition from an early age; others discovered its place in their lives only as adults; some have come to work with intuition only since learning Reiki. Yet all of these Reiki Masters appreciate the place of intuition in Reiki practice and understand that intuitive Reiki can act as a catalyst for deep and permanent healing.

GIFTED CHILD, GIFTED HEALER: LAURELLE SHANTI GAIA

Laurelle Shanti Gaia has been a student, a teacher, a practitioner, and a facilitator of the healing arts for more than thirty years. She served as a healer in the

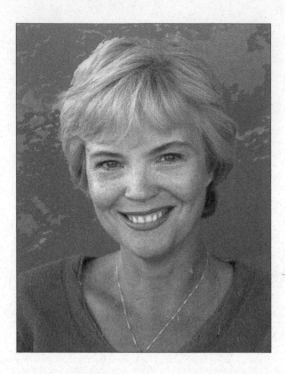

Laurelle Shanti Gaia

National Institute of Health's glioblastoma research project, a three-year study on the effects distant healing has on the quality of life for patients with this rare form of brain cancer. As a licensed Reiki Master and Karuna Reiki Master, she operates an active Reiki practice in Sedona, Arizona, where she founded the Infinite Light Healing Studies Center. Laurelle facilitates Reiki training programs in Sedona and worldwide.

Laurelle has written *Infinite Spectrum Color Healing Course, Sacred Circles, Be Peace Now,* and *The Book on Karuna Reiki.* These books and courses help students further understand and develop their subtle energy systems and soul-level chakras. Since 1994, Laurelle has served as director of teacher licensing for the International Center for Reiki Training. Laurelle also cofounded and facilitates the International Reiki Retreat in upstate New York and the Reiki and Sound Healing Conference in Sedona, Arizona.

Q: When did you first realize that you had some degree of natural intuitive ability? Did you welcome it or resist it?

A: I recall conversing with spiritual beings in my sandbox when I was about three years old. Also at age three, at Christmas time, my mother and I were using Glass Wax to stencil snowflakes and winter scenes on our windows. When we were finished I picked up a blue crayon and began to draw an image on the window. My mother asked who it was. I replied, "It's Mary."

"Mary WHO?" mother asked.

I replied, "You know, Mary, God's girl."

This was interesting because I was raised Lutheran. Most of the focus in Bible study was on Jesus; the Divine Mother was practically ignored. At age three I had virtually no experience in church. However, the Divine Mother would visit with me in a very playful way. I *knew* who she was.

I welcomed this ability and actually thought it was normal. I still do believe it is quite normal and that everyone has these abilities. They simply need to learn to remove the obstacles that some have created as a result of society's conditioning.

Q: What led you to Reiki? Did intuition or synchronicity play any part?

A: I knew at a very young age that I was called to the planet at this time to do healing work. When I was eight years old I decided it was time to become a responsible person, and of course responsible people have a plan for their lives. So I began to wonder what I should do with my life. Coincidentally, my grandmother had just given me a Bible. She said, "Honey, if you ever have any questions about life, all the answers are in this book." I thought this was wonderful. I would just look in this book and find out what I would do when I grew up.

As I diligently searched the Bible for the answer to my question, I became mesmerized by the stories of Jesus doing healing. I proudly announced to my family, "When I grow up, I am going to travel around the world and help heal people, and teach them that they can do this too."

The response was, "That's very nice, honey, but you can't do that, only Jesus can."

"Oh no," I said, "It says right here, 'He that believeth on me, the works that I do shall he do also; and greater works than these shall he do . . .'" [John 14:12].

"I know that's what it says, but that's not what it means," was the reply.

So for various reasons I allowed my inner knowing of my life's purpose to be blocked when I was just eight years old—but not before I had a little conversation with God. I said, "God, I really want to help people like Jesus did and they say I can't, but the Bible says I can. So I guess if I am supposed to do this, you'll figure it out and show me someday."

That prayer was completely released and forgotten, but looking back I'd say that I was guided from that moment on by a series of events and synchronicities. I was guided through good times and tough times. Sometimes I made the easy choice, and sometimes I made harder ones. But somehow God helped me find my way to live the answer to the prayer of an eight year old with a dream.

Q: Can you recall an early experience with intuition?

A: I am not certain this was my first experience, but it was quite memorable. One of the life experiences that led me to Reiki was observing my maternal grandfather, Grandpa John, battle with multiple sclerosis. The situation seemed so hopeless. Western medicine was unable to explain why he was ill. I promised my grandfather that someday I would find something that could help people who have multiple sclerosis and other serious illnesses. I believe that my statement of that intention, while connected with so much emotion, was one of the catalysts that propelled me along this path.

When I was thirteen years old, Grandpa John died. I was in the chapel at our church with my mother, brother, and sister. I saw Grandpa appear in the front left corner of the chapel. He was standing tall, and he looked so healthy. He was silent, but he had a beautiful smile. Then, in my mind's eye, I saw my father walking up the sidewalk on the side of the church. I turned to my mother and said, "Grandpa died and daddy is outside. He has come to get us."

My mother looked at me and asked, "What do you mean?"

I repeated myself and took my mother's hand and pulled her outside, insisting that we had to leave. As soon as we stepped outside, we met my father, who had indeed come to take us to my grandmother.

Q: How did you respond to this experience? Did you feel comfortable or

uncomfortable with this ability? Did the adults around you support or discourage this ability?

A: I was totally comfortable with this ability. It seemed very natural. The adults in my life usually tried to ignore it because they were uncomfortable with it. I do recall one conversation in which I was told that there is an imaginary world and a real world, and that I should stop talking about "these things" because people would think there is something wrong with me.

Q: How long ago were you attuned to Reiki and by whom?

A: My first "official" attunement was sixteen years ago, by Karen Patton. However, I had two rather profound spiritual experiences at the age of eight. When I reflect back on those experiences, what I felt was quite similar to a Reiki initiation attunement. I have often wondered if I somehow received spontaneous attunements during those experiences. Immediately after both incidents, I felt a stronger energy flowing through me. When I finally received my first "official" attunement, I didn't feel any particular energetic change at all and was actually a little disappointed. However, I was more confident after that attunement, and began to immediately focus on Reiki and healing for myself and others.

> *Laurelle doesn't remember her Reiki Master mentioning to her that she might experience an increase in her intuitive abilities as she practiced Reiki, nor does she feel that Reiki caused any immediate increase in her intuitive abilities. She does acknowledge that all her "spiritual sensory abilities" have increased "over time" and that her intuition has become even more helpful.*

Q: As a newly attuned practitioner, were you able to recognize the value of intuitive impressions received while doing Reiki and offer them to help your clients discover their healing purpose?

A: I was a little hesitant at first, because some of the impressions seemed odd or illogical. Also, I believe I had a little of that old audiotape playing in my head reminding me that I should not talk about "these things," because "people might think there is something wrong with me." However, I realized at one point that my hesitation was personality or ego-based, and that it was interfering. So I learned to begin each session with a prayer of intention, which included giving thanks that "my personality and ego stand aside so that I am a completely clear channel for the Reiki energy to work through." After I started doing this, the impressions were clearer, and I shared them freely, and I was not attached to a client's acceptance or to the outcome in any way.

Q: When you teach Reiki now, do you let your students know that intuition will be enhanced? Do you provide them with any instruction in how to work with it?

A: I do mention that all their spiritual sensory abilities may be enhanced. I teach how to use intuition to determine where to direct Reiki energy, but I don't go into this in depth. I do not believe that having a keen awareness of one's intuition is necessary for a person to begin to practice Reiki. Many beginning students don't believe they have intuition, or they don't trust their intuition. So I want those students to be confident that they, too, will be able to practice Reiki. Therefore, I don't place a lot of emphasis on intuition. In the more advanced classes this is addressed in more detail, and I teach some visualization exercises and some techniques that a person can practice, which often result in increased intuitive abilities.

Q: Can you give an example of how intuition has supported you as you gave a Reiki treatment?

A: Although I do not diagnose illness, my intuition has "told" me from time to time that a client has a specific illness. There was one particular instance in which I was scanning a woman's aura to assess her energy. As my hand passed about six inches above her abdominal area I literally heard the words *liver cancer*. I didn't tell her what I heard. I continued with a basic Reiki treatment. At the end of the session I told her that I felt an imbalance in her abdominal area, and that after the treatment it felt a little clearer, but I encouraged her to see her physician. She telephoned a few days later and told me she had been diagnosed with liver cancer and was scheduled for surgery. Half of her liver was removed in the surgery. She returned to me post-surgery and received Reiki several more times. Over the course of a few months of regular Reiki treatments, her liver regenerated, and she was told she was completely cancer free.

Q: Have you any comments or suggestions for those Reiki practitioners who would like to become more intuitively guided in their practice?

A: Invoke the Reiki energy, pray for guidance, act on the guidance, let go of expectation, and trust that the outcome will always serve the highest good. Also, expand your awareness. Your intuition can "speak" to you in a multitude of ways. You may have visions, hear messages, simply have an inner knowing—or other people may say something that brings wisdom to you that you have been seeking. The universe is vast, as are the many ways that your intuition can communicate.

I believe the most important skill a person interested in healing or expanding intuition can develop is the ability to listen. You cannot be aware of intuitive messages if you are always talking or thinking. Practice giving one hundred percent of your attention to anyone who speaks to you, and really *listen*. Multi-tasking is not supportive of intuitive development, but stillness is. I believe that our intuition is our direct connection with Divine consciousness, and it is within the stillness that we can truly be aware of this connection. During Reiki sessions I often remember to "Be still and know that I am God" [Psalm 46:10].

INTUITIVE AWARENESS OF THE POWER OF PRAYER: WILLIAM LEE RAND

William Lee Rand, founder and president of The International Center for Reiki Training, is the author of three books: *Reiki: The Healing Touch*, *Reiki for a New Millennium*, and, with Frank Arjava Petter and Walter Lubeck, *The Spirit of Reiki*. He is also editor in chief of the *Reiki News Magazine*, editor of the *Online Reiki Newsletter*, and the author of many articles and tapes on Reiki. In 1997 he traveled to the North Pole; in 1999, to the South Pole; and in 2004, to Jerusalem, to place world peace grids at these locations as focal points for meditations and Reiki distant healing.

William was attuned and certified as a Reiki I and II practitioner in 1981 and

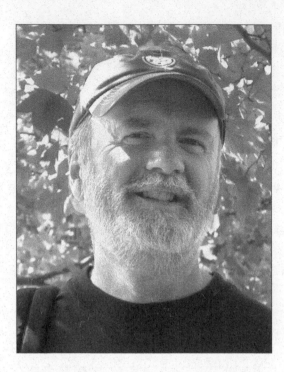

William Lee Rand

1982 by Bethel Phaigh, a Reiki Master trained by Hawayo Takata. He studied the Reiki Master course of training first with Diane McCumber in 1989, and later with four other Reiki masters: Marlene Schilke, Leah Smith, Hiroshi Doi, and Hyakuten Inamoto. He has traveled to Japan many times to do research on Reiki.

Q: Can you recall your first experience with intuition, either your own or someone else's?

A: I have lots of experiences with intuition now, as an adult, but remembering the first one as a child? I can't. My intuition did become much stronger to me when I started doing meditation and studying metaphysics. Before that, it wasn't quite as pronounced.

I will tell you about one experience with my mother. I must have been nine years old when this happened. She lost the car keys, and she was worried that my father would be upset with her. She got into the backseat and she prayed and asked for guidance—and right away she found the keys. It worked! That experience, maybe because it was with my mother, gave me a connection to an energy and to divine guidance that I hadn't noticed before. I could feel something in my mother's consciousness that opened—a trust, belief in a higher power. I saw her ask and pray, and this gave me an awareness of intuition, an internal experience of the energy, the shift in consciousness that took place in my mother. I could feel it. Maybe that was one of my first experiences of the divine, or maybe it was an altered state. There was also a feeling of humility and of sacredness in that moment.

Q: How did you respond to this experience? Did you feel comfortable with it?

A: I saw how she did it, and thought I could use that. The fact that it did something meaningful and had an immediate result—helped her find the car keys—had an impact. I could see the relationship between cause and effect, how her asking for guidance, praying, opening to receive, worked. It wasn't like most prayers. There was a real opening in her consciousness.

Q: Is this when you first realized that you had some degree of natural intuitive ability? Did you welcome it?

A: Yes, I welcomed it. I thought I could use it, too.

Q: What led you to Reiki? Did intuition or synchronicity play any part?

A: I first found out about Reiki at a week-long rebirthing training seminar in 1981. Bethel Phaigh just happened to be there and she offered to talk about Reiki. I had been raised as a Christian. I started reading the Bible at an early age, especially about Jesus's miracles and healing. I also started studying metaphysics in high school, and I realized there was a connection between them, but the people at the church discouraged me from thinking that and, as a result, I drifted away from the church. One of the things that Bethel said right away about Reiki was that this was similar to the healing that Jesus did, and that was exactly what I wanted to find. It fit.

Q: Did Bethel Phaigh, who taught you Reiki I and II, tell you to expect an increase or enhancement in your intuitive abilities?

A: Yes, she did. I remember she told us that Takata said "Once you have Reiki, your Reiki hands will guide you." After you've done a complete treatment you can go back and do more healing, and your Reiki hands will guide you to the right places.

Bethel also said that Reiki connects you much more strongly to Source or the higher power, and that your whole life will be guided by intuition, and you can more easily be guided to your spiritual purpose. That was significant for me. I decided after taking level II to really focus on finding my life purpose. And I began saying a prayer: "Guide me and heal me so that I may be of greater service to others." I don't how many times I've said that prayer. I began saying that prayer and my life changed. That was when my life shifted. Prior to that, I hadn't really been living a life that was guided by intuition or by the higher power. I was planning to stay in Hawaii my whole life but I found myself coming back to Detroit. It turned out to be the right place to be, even though, intellectually, I never would have come back to Detroit. I just took one guided step after another, and things just kept getting better. I kept asking for guidance and then taking the next step. I continue to do this today.

Q: Did Bethel Phaigh provide you with any instruction in how to work with your intuition when impressions came up while you did Reiki?

A: No, but she did say that the best place to do Reiki on a client isn't necessarily the most logical. If you treat an area that seems logical and it doesn't seem to be working, ask for guidance on where to put your hands. I worked on a client who had a hip problem, but when I worked on her hips, I didn't feel much going on there. I asked for guidance, and I was directed to work on her knees. That helped her.

Q: Once you were attuned to Reiki, did you notice an immediate increase in your intuitive abilities, or was this a skill that developed with practice?

A: I feel Reiki did increase my intuition, but using intention and saying prayer really increased it. Knowing that Reiki increased my intuition encouraged me to use my intention and ask for guidance and then seek to follow it.

Q: When you teach Reiki, do you let your students know that intuition will be enhanced?

A: Yes, I tell them it will. I explain how to use intuition when I teach scanning and Reiji-ho. I also remind them to value intuition generally. I say, "Let yourselves be guided in where to put your hands, what symbols to use, what techniques to use." I want them to know that asking for guidance can be very helpful.

Q: Have you any comments or suggestions you would like to make to those Reiki practitioners who would like to become more intuitively guided in their practice?

A: Just trust. Even if you think it is just your imagination, try it. Trust in the Reiki energy and follow your impressions. That will really help you to develop your intuitive skill.

DREAMWORKER: ROBERT FUESTON

Reiki Master Robert Fueston started practicing Reiki in 1996 and teaching in 1997. In 1999, while working in a medical library and completing his master's degree in library and information science, he decided to pursue a career in Chinese medicine. Robert used his learning as a librarian to research the origins of Reiki. This inevitably led him into finding, conversing, and training with some of the remaining twenty-two Reiki Master students of Hawayo Takata. Aspects of this research can be found in *The Reiki Sourcebook* by Frans and Bronwen Stiene and on his website, www.robertfueston.com.

Before responding to any of my questions, Robert offered a definition of *intuition* in order to make clear the fact that he does not "take on" his clients' imbalances. Here is what Robert said.

"Intuition can occur on many levels. There are a variety of ways that Reiki communicates with practitioners. A practitioner may 'hear' messages, may feel in his or her own body where problems are in the client's body, may just sense the area of imbalance in the client's body, et cetera. Having these experiences does not mean that the practitioner is taking on the client's imbalances. Rather, it is just the way Reiki is communicating to the practitioner what needs to be addressed and where to go with the hands for the treatment."

Q: When did you first realize that you had some degree of natural intuitive ability? Did you welcome it or resist it?

A: When I was in kindergarten or first grade I had a dream one night that was a little too "different" from other dreams—it was one long story and it felt very real. The following night my dream picked up from where it had left off the night before. The next morning I told my parents what had happened. I told them that I couldn't wait until the night because I was interested in finding out how the "dream" would end. My parents told me dreams don't work that way. That night I went to sleep and dreamt the third and final part of the dream.

That experience was so fascinating to me, and still is. I have come to the conclusion that there are "junk" dreams, which mean nothing, and there are what I like to call "organic" dreams, which are meaningful and may not be dreams at all. These are real experiences that your spirit is having somewhere other than here on Earth—possibly in a different realm/dimension/time. Later, during my formal training in Chinese medicine, I discovered that this sort of thing occurs by virtue of the spirit of the organs.

Q: Can you recall your first experience with intuition, either your own or someone else's?

A: When I was in seventh grade I had a dream one night; the next morning I saw the event from my dream occur in waking life. The event took place for only ten seconds or so, but it was a strange phenomenon to experience.

Q: How did you respond to this experience? Did you feel comfortable or uncomfortable with this ability? Did the adults around you support or discourage this ability?

A: At that age I just thought it was weird. I don't remember if I shared it with my parents or not. If I did share it, I cannot remember their response.

Q: Did intuition play any part in your journey to Reiki?

A: Yes, intuition and divine presence played a role in my Reiki journey. I had bought a Reiki book through One Spirit book club. The book sat on my shelf for over a year before I even picked it up. One day, out of the blue, I decided to read the introduction. It sounded interesting, but I figured that since you had to be taught Reiki by a teacher, there was little chance of me meeting one where I lived. Later that week I was in a café and noticed a flyer advertising a Reiki class. I immediately called the teacher and was told that I would have to set up a class for him to teach, which I did. I have been practicing ever since. My first Reiki class was on October 28, 1996, by a man named Anthony Thiebaut, who went by the name of Spirit. I have had several other Reiki teachers since then, including Jone Eagle, Light and Adonea, Hiroshi Doi, Hyakuten Inamoto, and two of Takata's masters, John Harvey Gray and Fran Brown.

Q: Has your intuition become stronger and more helpful since you learned Reiki?

A: Absolutely! I feel that the practice of Reiki keeps us more connected to the "all"—Source, God, Creator, Tao, whatever you want to call it. The stronger your connection, the more "supernatural" senses, such as intuition, become plainly natural. Reiki is simply one way of strengthening your connection to the "all."

Q: When you teach Reiki do you let your students know that intuition will be enhanced? Do you provide them with any instruction in how to work with it?

A: When the timing is right I tell students that their intuition will probably develop with the practice of Reiki. It may not be in the class that I tell them this. I have a Reikishare for my students each week where we share Reiki stories and treatments and I "teach" through stories and examples about Reiki.

I think that once a student recognizes that the teacher's intuition is keen, then the student is able to develop intuition even faster. Seeing that it can be done greatly enhances the belief that it is possible to do. Part of the problem for students is that they will intuit things but they don't trust their intuition. This is where having an encouraging teacher may help.

Q: Would you please share a story of how you first experienced your intuition as you treated a client—or yourself—with Reiki?

A: One of my first experiences of intuition during a treatment occurred when I was treating the back of a young woman, and I suddenly started to feel a lot of anger. The emotion was interesting to me. I was feeling anger but I wasn't really angry about anything. After the treatment the young woman asked me if I picked up on anything. Since I was relatively new to Reiki, I didn't feel comfortable telling her exactly what I felt. So I simply mentioned that her lower back took a lot of Reiki. She was amazed and commented that when I was treating her lower back she felt anger rise up in her, as she had started to think of some personal issues that were going on for her.

When these types of situations arise repeatedly, you learn to trust your intuition. Although at the time I didn't know it, this experience would reflect my future Reiki experiences with intuition. For example, once during a Reiki client treatment I experienced an uncomfortable feeling, and then the word *work* popped into my head. My client mentioned that she was no longer satisfied with her work situation and was planning on changing jobs. She had only told a few people about this and didn't want her employer to find out yet.

Q: Would you please share a story of how intuition works to support Reiki healing when you do treatments now?

A: I think that using Reiki and having the ability to connect with someone using intuition helps with the person's healing. It might be as simple as being able to pick up on a site where the client has previously broken a bone, for example. On a more immediate level, when working with a client who is going through a mental/emotional upset or is contemplating a major change in life or career, the ability to bring the issue up first usually astonishes the person, but in a way that makes the person feel that it is okay to discuss the issue with you. It is not the job of a Reiki practitioner to give advice, but the practitioner can do the treatment and be a good listener. This is sometimes enough for the client to work it out for himself or herself.

Q: Has Reiki practice helped you to evolve into a more intuitive person?

A: Absolutely. I have a slogan: "Intuition—don't leave home without it."

CROSSING BORDERS, BRINGING HEALING, TEACHING PEACE: MARI HALL

American Reiki Master Mari Hall was the first to teach Reiki in the United Kingdom, Norway, and Czechoslovakia, and one of the first to bring Reiki to the European Union. President Vaclev Havel of the Czech Republic recognized this work when Mari was nominated for the prestigious Heart of the Country award, which is the Czech equivalent to the Nobel Peace Prize. Mari, who is the Founding Director of the International Association of Reiki (established in 1989), works actively with the International Board of Complementary Medicine for the standardization of teaching and professional practice of Reiki within the European Union.

Mari has taught Reiki to over 45,000 people worldwide; she has also written several Reiki books, all international best sellers: *Practical Reiki, Reiki for Common Ailments, Reiki for the Soul: Ten Doorways to Inner Peace,* and *Reiki: Using Healing Energy for Peace, Joy, and Vitality.* Mari cofounded and facilitates the semiannual twenty-one-day Virtual Usui Retreat.

Q: What led you to Reiki? Did intuition or synchronicity play any part?

A: Synchronicity played a big part. I was partially paralyzed and looking for an alternative to classical medicine. I was in a bookstore looking at yet another self-help book when a woman I barely knew came up to me and hugged me. First of all, I wasn't huggable, and the most astonishing thing was that I could feel her hands on me hours later. When I called her to ask what she did to me other than the hug, she said it must be Reiki. I took a course the next week, and the rest is history. Reiki found me.

Q: Can you recall your first experience with intuition, either your own or someone else's? How did you respond to this experience?

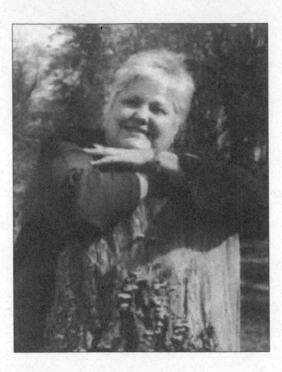

Mari Hall

A: I was always intuitive, even as a child. I knew of things that were going to happen, I saw things that adults did not, but I started to question my gift in puberty; after Reiki I trusted more what was always there.

I was always comfortable with my insight. It was part of me as a child so I thought it was natural. I always welcomed it, but I wanted to know why I had "it" when others did not. It was an escape when things were too bad at home. I was off with the fairies or busy seeing levels of things.

> *Mari was attuned to Reiki by Iris Ishikuro, one of the Reiki Masters trained by Hawayo Takata, in 1980. She was told to expect an increase in her intuitive abilities but was not provided with any specific instruction, because, Mari says, her teacher "realized I had been this way and needed no help."*

Q: Once you were attuned to Reiki did you notice an immediate increase in your intuitive abilities, or was this a skill that developed with practice?

A: I would say that I noticed an immediate increase, and then as I came into the practice my intuition was heightened.

Q: As a newly attuned practitioner, were you able to recognize the value of intuitive impressions received while doing Reiki and offer them to help your clients discover their healing purpose?

A: Yes, but I do not impose what I see on them. I may gently question. It is important for me that they have a realization and not that I have one for them.

Q: Has your intuition become stronger and more helpful since you learned Reiki?

A: Yes, very much so.

Q: When you teach Reiki, do you let your students know that intuition will be enhanced? Do you provide them with any instruction in how to work with it?

A: Yes, I do, and if they ask I tell them. I do not emphasize this. Rather, I work with them to trust their hands and what they feel. Of course, this is intuitive.

Q: Can you give me an example of how intuition has supported you in interactions with a student or as you offered a Reiki treatment?

A: I always get a read on a student, and usually, in the course of conversation, things come forward that validate what I "knew." Also, when treating, I am aware of how I feel inside myself. Once I touch the client I immediately feel inside me where to place my hands. I have worked with thousands of people in clinical application. I trust my hands.

Q: Have you any comments or suggestions you would like to make to those Reiki practitioners who would like to become more intuitively guided in their practice?

A: Practice, practice, and practice some more. Be still inside. The moment you lose your demand to be more of anything and accept where you are in this moment, you move into *now*, and this space is where pure insight springs from. Let it move with you. It is not a mind thing. It is a living experience.

Q: Is there anything further you would like to add?

A: Reiki is a spiritual practice that takes time. It is a journey, not a destination. Enjoy the journey, and allow it to take you slowly and softly in the flow. The practice of Reiki is the most important factor. Use the energy for oneself and others daily.

GROUNDED PRACTICE, GUIDED EARTH STEWARDSHIP: JANEANNE NARRIN

janeAnne Narrin is the author of *One Degree Beyond: A Reiki Journey into Energy Medicine*, which won the Coalition of Visionary Retailers' "Visionary Award" in the alternative health category; she is also the author of several books of poetry and nonfiction and a website based on whole-systems theory (see www. webpages.charter.net/jtnarrin/). A resident of Asheville, North Carolina, jane-Anne is a longtime Reiki Master and is cofounder and past facilitator of the semiannual twenty-one-day Virtual Usui Retreat. A former corporate consultant, janeAnne now serves as a broker and realtor to create private trusts for the preservation of beautiful wilderness lands. Her focus on stewardship of wilderness lands, sustainability, and healthy-built homes emerges out of a passionate commitment to healing the Earth, beginning at home.

Q. Can you recall your first experience with intuition, either your own or someone else's?

A: When I was a child my life was rich with extraordinary experiences. My first experience with intuition had to do with my grandmother's favorite brooch, a cameo her mother had given her when she was only twelve. It was just a small piece, but I sensed that it had vast import to Grandma, and so I asked her to tell me the story of how it came to mean so much to her. She seemed to heal somehow with that acknowledgement.

Q: When did you first realize that you had some degree of natural intuitive ability? Did you welcome it or resist it?

A: I must have been four or five. I welcomed it.

Q: What part did intuition play in your journey to Reiki, if any?

A: Intuition was the key to my journey into Reiki and into the practice of Reiki. As I recount in my book, *One Degree Beyond: A Reiki Journey into Energy Medicine,* "I made myself the promise to be open to opportunity and to be willing to follow the signposts along the way." Looking back now after almost twenty years, I realize that, by honoring my choice to let intuition guide me, I discovered energy of pure potential—a simultaneous coming together and a letting go. I reaped the reward of that choice.

> *janeAnne's willingness to reflect on her own soul's journey and to value the guidance she received enabled her "to understand how trusting process, in concert with paying attention, leads to a new level of perception and awakening." This helped to create a new sense of order and balance within that was soon reflected in her 'outer' life. She adds, "What a joy it is to discover that, when you relinquish that which you prize, things of even greater significance appear."*

Q: How long ago were you attuned to Reiki and by whom?

A: I was attuned almost twenty years ago, in a cabin in which Takata herself taught on Orcas Island, north of Seattle. It felt as if her energy was present on the days that I spent learning from a Reiki teacher whose own teacher was Takata's granddaughter, Phyllis Furumoto.

> *While this Reiki Master mentioned that janeAnne might experience an increase in her intuitive abilities as a result of being attuned to Reiki, she was not given any specific instruction in how to work with intuitive impressions in the Reiki I class; this was given as part of the advanced Reiki training. She notes, "As for how to work with intuition when impressions come up, we were instructed to be very careful about this, as such perceptions can be seductive to the ego, especially for new initiates in the practice. Many times the newly initiated are enthusiastic about 'intuitions' that arise. It is pretty exciting for them, but experience teaches patience. My Reiki teachers taught me to first release my attachment to what I think the outcome or*

healing effect should be; and second, to trust Reiki. Such a simple formula for success!"

Unlike most practitioners, who study Reiki with only one or two teachers, janeAnne had the extraordinary good fortune to meet and learn from many of the original twenty-two Reiki Masters Takata herself taught. "They have been my mentors. Instruction came to me as I came to understand the meanings of their stories. I learned through stories and through my experience with the practice of Reiki. So I learned 'intuitively.'" All of janeAnne's teachers emphasized the importance of "paying attention and staying present" while doing Reiki self-treatment and client treatment. This allows deeper understanding to emerge.

Q: Once you were attuned to Reiki did you notice an immediate increase in your intuitive abilities, or was this a skill that developed with practice?

A: Actually, I noticed an integration of my intuitive skills into a whole system of being in the moment within a process for wellness.

Q: As a newly attuned practitioner, were you able to recognize the value of intuitive impressions received while doing Reiki and offer them to help your clients discover their healing purpose?

A: In the very strict First Degree [Reiki I] training, the newly initiated are cautioned *not* to share impressions, because we are neophytes in energy work. At this level, initiates are encouraged to look within and use their intuition to "first heal yourself," as Takata recommended. So unless you are without ego, the advice is to be respectful of Reiki, where all intuition flows without words.

Q: Has your intuition become stronger and more helpful since you learned Reiki?

A: It feels to me as comfortable as the changing leaves in autumn—something upon which I simply can rely, part of an ongoing process to which I can choose to attend. It has been my friend more and more as I journey through life. And, yes, daily practice of Reiki over almost twenty years certainly enhances the connection, and that is helpful.

Although a highly experienced practitioner and teacher, janeAnne still feels reluctant to share her impressions of "the hows and whys of wellness for another." For this reason, at the beginning of a Reiki treatment she prays and sets her intention that whatever impressions emerge during the session come into the client's mind, rather than her own. If the client feels inclined to share these impressions, she will listen with complete attention and compassion.

Q: When you teach Reiki, do you let your students know that intuition will be enhanced? Do you provide them with any instruction in how to work with it?

A: I tell them the stories: of Dr. Usui, his journey, his intuitions; of Hayashi, his journey, his intuitions; of Takata, her journey, her intuitions; of the "miracles of healing" throughout history. Then I ask them what the stories mean. We talk about how so much potential may open up for them as they practice Reiki. It may express itself as art forms, as insight, as a joyful heart, as a way to create space in the world for the healing of Mother Earth herself.

I require students to focus first on healing what needs to be healed within, and to let this be the intent. Should enhanced intuition unfold because they are dedicated to the practice of Reiki, I know they will work on advanced training. At that point, side by side we will explore how Reiki manifests in their lives, and how intuition plays a role in the whole process.

I stress the absolute importance of satisfying the requirement of being able to release attachment to outcome. I suggest that approaching their practice for others with as little ego as possible is to be desired. Over the past many years I have come to see that only the very few "angels of Reiki on Earth" can say that there is no agenda, whether conscious or not, behind what they may offer to another intuitively. Many students have to admit that offering intuitive insights to others makes them feel good about themselves and very powerful—and so it comes down to them; whereas the practice of Reiki for others is about unselfishly connecting as a channel for wellness.

Q: Would you please share a story of how you first experienced your intuition as you treated a client—or yourself—with Reiki?

A: Before Reiki is drawn by a client in a Reiki session, I remind myself to trust the intelligence that *is* Reiki. After all, I remind myself, Reiki is "on the job" bringing expanded awareness with it. So "just for today," I can relax, not worry, and stay out of the way. Respectfully, at the start and after the session, I may ask my clients to pay particular attention to any "sense" that may arise.

In my daily practice, often I am aware of physical releases/sensations that speak to me of healing. Mostly, I pay attention to what my body is telling me and correct my trajectory—although I still seem to love chocolate, sometimes too much.

Q: Would you please share a story of how intuition works to support Reiki healing when you do treatments now?

A: I can share a story, but it is about how intuition and Reiki go hand-in-hand *outside* the individual and client-based practice of Reiki. It is the story of following your heart to new places and ways of being in the world.

A few years back the stories of my childhood and my intuition led me to another adventure. For some reason, James Taylor's song "In My Mind I'm Going to Carolina," kept playing over and over in my head. The song was the harbinger. Family matters and history led me to "come home" to Asheville, where I landed with an open heart and willingness to contribute in a positive way. I opened Spirit Ridge, a center for wellness, and Reiki flowed. But something else was happening. Each day during Reiki [self-treatment], the spirit of the Appalachians seemed to reach out to me. Was it time for my Reiki practice to embrace the larger community? Possibly so, for within a short time my devotion to stewardship of old Appalachian farmlands and mountain terrains blossomed.

Q: Has Reiki practice helped you to evolve into a more intuitive person?

A: It seems to me that devotion over a period of years to daily Reiki practice helps each of us to manifest wonderful things, including increased levels of awareness and intuition. One thing is for sure: I know that the point of it all is to let go of expecting things to work out just the way you think they should (they rarely do anyway!), and to bring your best self to each situation you encounter in your life while awakening kindness at every chance you get.

PROFESSIONAL INTUITIVE READER
AND LIGHTWORKER: LINDA SCHILLER-HANNA

Linda Schiller-Hanna is a professional intuitive who has read more than twenty thousand people worldwide and taught more than one thousand students in her Lightworker Intensive course. She lectures with the Association for Research and Enlightenment on intuition development nationwide and will soon launch an internet radio station (www.lightworker22radio.com). Linda founded Angel Love Healing Center, which is especially involved in helping people with AIDS. She has been a Reiki Master for nearly ten years and feels that Reiki and intuition are twin sources of joy in her life.

Q: When did you first realize that you had some degree of natural intuitive ability? Did you welcome it or resist it?

A: I had a lot of "random" hits for many years. I'd think of someone, the phone would ring, and it would be that person. Most people have these kind of events. I always thought it was neat, but felt there was no way I could get better at it or learn to do it on demand. I just thought I had a "bit" of psychic ability. Whenever it happened, I felt a private thrill, a secret joy.

Q: Can you recall your first experience with intuition, either your own or someone else's?

A: Yes, I was living in Vallejo, California. My brother Joe was staying with us and he and I always shared a fascination with all things mysterious and psychic. One afternoon we were playing with a deck of cards. He suggested that we practice telepathy. Joe would look at the cards one by one, and I was to receive, letting him know if they were red or black. I actually wasn't doing too well with this game, mainly because I was trying too hard. However, in the middle of the game I had a sudden impression that came through strongly. I stopped the game and wrote it down.

My husband was in the Navy at the time, and he had recently been transferred from the USS Forrestal to Mare Island. We had a friend still stationed on the ship whom I knew to be on a vacation in the Mediterranean. I suddenly thought

257

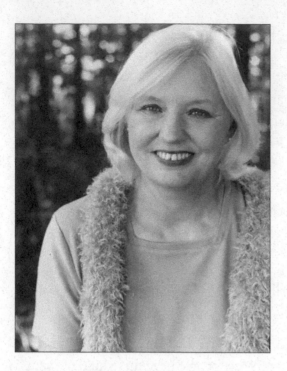

Linda Schiller-Hanna

of our friend Chuck and felt he was standing on a hill, looking out to sea and thinking about me. I wrote him a letter and he answered back, confirming that at that very time he was actually doing this. We knew there were at least five thousand miles between us.

Q: How did you respond to this experience? Did you feel comfortable or uncomfortable with this ability?

A: I was quite amazed by it. My brother enjoyed it, our friend Chuck was also amazed, and my husband shrugged it off. I don't think a lot of attention was paid to it; it seemed more "coincidental" than anything. But the experience continued to rumble around in the back of my mind and I began to read more and more about psychics and other metaphysical topics.

Q: What led you to Reiki? Did intuition or synchronicity play any part?

A: I first learned of Reiki from Penny Price, a Reiki healer and TV producer with the *Merv Griffin Show,* whom I had as a guest on my cable TV show, *The Natural Psychic,* in Los Angeles in 1984. It was my sixteenth show, with the topic of the

258

third chakra and power. Penny introduced me to Reiki and was an eloquent spokeswoman for its usage. She was an advanced Reiki practitioner at the time, and she shared a miraculous story about Reiki helping heal a burn very swiftly. I remember being very impressed and thinking, "Someday I want to learn to do that, too."

I first experienced a Reiki treatment from my friend Sandra Barraza, in Mazatlan, Mexico, around 1986. She had taken Reiki I and wanted to show me what it was like. Sandra had done energetic treatments before she learned Reiki and was very good at those, but I felt a definite difference in what she offered now that she was opened with Reiki. I felt that the energy was warmer, stronger, more vibrant than other healing treatments I'd experienced from her, or anyone else for that matter.

There is a funny story about how I actually found my first Reiki teacher. I was living in Virginia Beach and had used a local holistic newspaper to line one of my drawers. Doris Denby, a local Reiki Master with top lineage, had an article in the paper, and her face greeted me every morning when I opened the drawer. After a few months of this, I felt her speak telepathically to me, saying "It's time for you to come learn from me." So I did. I was attuned December 11, 1992. My second Reiki Master was Joseph Nicely. I took Reiki II with him about two years later. My teacher for the Reiki Master course was Eleanor Perkins; I took that course in 1996 in Cuyahoga Falls, Ohio.

Q: Did the Reiki Master who first attuned you tell you to expect an increase or enhancement in your intuitive abilities?

A: There were two of us in my class, Anna Lee Scully and myself. Anna Lee was a graduate of my Lightworker Intensive already, so we were both open channels, and Doris Denby knew this. I don't remember it coming up, because we were already quite open.

Q: Once you were attuned to Reiki, did you notice an immediate increase in your intuitive abilities, or was this a skill that developed with practice?

A: I developed my psychic abilities in 1979 and 1980 at a school in Berkeley, California, called Heartsong. I was working professionally at least ten years before I learned Reiki, so intuition came first for me. What I did notice, however, was a huge and powerful cleansing after taking Reiki II. I refer to it as my "crash and burn" days. My whole world fell apart at that time, and I had to leave behind many useless and cherished icons of an unenlightened consciousness. During those days I released my patterns of victimhood and of attracting abusive men and I let go of hand-to-mouth financial attitudes, of hating my parents, and of other useless emotional baggage. I went through a period of paranoia, went two months without having a real home, and other freaky experiences.

Suffice it to say that the cleansing was necessary and as brutal as it needed to be for me to let go of blockages that didn't allow my higher self to flow freely into action, whether for healing or intuitive counseling work. It wasn't pretty, and I'm glad it's over. I don't miss one iota of the garbage I dumped from those painful days. I feel that Reiki II was a direct catalyst for that transformation. Maybe it was inevitable, but I see these events as a seamless process.

Since I became a Reiki Master, my whole life has blossomed.

Q: As a newly attuned practitioner, were you able to recognize the value of intuitive impressions received while doing Reiki and offer them to help your client discover their healing purpose?

A: Since being trained at Heartsong in 1979 and 1980, I have always valued my intuitive impressions. I use them both for counseling and healing purposes. I couldn't be a healer without my intuition being active. It would be like driving a car with no engine! I am not a true Reiki purist, which is one of the reasons I don't teach Reiki. I am so busy combining my impressions, counseling tools, and so on into the process that Reiki may be only fifty percent of what I am offering at the moment. I feel I offer a hybrid form of Reiki in most cases.

Q: Has your intuition become stronger and more helpful since you learned Reiki?

A: My intuition becomes clearer and brighter each year. Reiki and all the other things I do to heal my life are all part of that clarity. I can't imagine myself without the use of my intuition or my Reiki skills. They are like the right and left chambers of my heart.

Q: When you teach Reiki do you let your students know that intuition will be enhanced? Do you provide them with any instruction in how to work with it?

A: I don't teach Reiki. I have my hands full teaching intuition, and there are many others who do teach Reiki quite excellently. I have so deeply integrated Reiki into my life that I don't feel I could articulate it. It's something I am, rather than something I know. To teach Reiki would be like trying to stop my autonomic nervous system and break it down into tiny steps. I don't think in those terms.

My Reiki II teacher, Joe Nicely, covered intuition quite extensively in his course. He had already taken my Lightworker course, however. There was quite a bit of overlapping information.

I have a learning disability and believe that I amassed Reiki awareness on a more subconscious level rather than a conscious level. I feel that in most of my Reiki classes I was in an altered state. That's another reason I can't teach it.

Q: Can you give an example of how intuition has supported you as you offered Reiki treatment or interacted with a student?

A: About 1994, shortly after I learned Reiki II, a friend of mine had a serious car accident in which her lungs collapsed. The doctors were able to get one side up and working and then the other, but she was not allowed to leave the hospital until both lungs were stabilized. I worked with Heather daily using Reiki, and she made slow improvements. But there were disappointing relapses. One lung would work awhile and then go down again. The other would come on line and then it, too, would collapse.

Heather is a healer, as are both of her parents. We are all Lightworkers. Although she was young and vibrant, she was just not making good progress. Near the end of the second week of her hospitalization, my guides whispered to me that we needed more help. They suggested that I ask Joe Nicely, my Reiki II teacher, to come and help give Reiki treatments at the hospital. I called him and he agreed, and he also brought his girlfriend, who is a Reiki practitioner. This time, three of us worked together on Heather's lungs. It seemed to go well.

The next day, the doctors reported that Heather's lungs were holding steady and that she could leave the hospital for further recovery at home. We were exultant!

Q: Can you give me an example of how receiving an intuitive impression as you treated yourself with Reiki has helped you?

A: It's often hard for me to think to give myself Reiki. I do it, especially if I fall or pull a muscle or experience a sudden injury. Many healers have difficulty with self-healing, I think. I have a lot of faith in God. When I am in pain I often forget the complex Reiki symbols. What I do most often is put both hands on the wound and silently say to myself: "Reiki, Reiki, Reiki" And that's about it. Then I will get some kind of impression of other ways I can help myself. As a Cayce follower, I may feel that I need to prepare a castor oil pack for a sprained ankle, or once, when I fell on the ice, I took an epsom salt bath. Each injury seems to bring forth different healing answers as required. All I know is, I always seem to get help. For most of the years I have done readings, and for five of the years I have known Reiki, I did not have medical insurance, but even with a variety of ailments and maladies, I have always gotten well.

Q: Have you any comments or suggestions you would like to make to those Reiki practitioners who would like to become more intuitively guided in their practice?

A: First of all, when you have committed to learning and doing Reiki, you are already one of God's healing angels. God is helping you in every possible way and certainly would not ask you to do this work without giving immediate and personalized guidance on the spot each and every time you serve. Assume it's there, and assume it's right, and use it accordingly.

I recommend that you work with your intuition on a regular basis. I encourage you to study with a teacher to become familiar with the nuances of the process. My Lightworker Intensive is a wonderful weekend course that gives a quick start to anyone wishing to learn. The Association for Research and Enlightenment has great intuition training programs, and there are others around the world. Basically, intuition is about consciousness. If there is too much "glamorous razzle dazzle" associated with the class and the teacher, it may be a clue that the teacher's motives are not as evolved as you really want. I encourage you to see a photo of the teacher and trust your own intuition to help you decide if this is the right person for you to open up with. If you have doubts, ask prospective teachers how they cover ethics in their class. By their fruits, you will know them.

Q: Is there anything further you would like to add?

A: I'd recommend that anyone who does Reiki read the list of Precepts of Miracles from the *Course in Miracles*. This is the first page of the teacher's manual. It makes a wonderful point: "There is no order of difficulty in miracles."

Be not afraid to address anything with Reiki. I have done Reiki on an airplane for a man who had an epileptic seizure. I have done it for a woman at the scene of a car accident, while she was shaking and being interviewed by a policeman. I wrapped a blanket around her as she shivered and secretly gave Reiki while holding the blanket.

I gave Reiki to three people in comas. Although the cases looked hopeless, all three emerged: one on the spot, one in a couple of days, and one—who I thought was on the way to the grave—went home well in a few weeks. Basically, just show up. Do what you do. Pray fervently. Don't see the illness; see the divine soul in front of you and love that soul.

Q: Has Reiki practice helped you to evolve into a more intuitive person?

A: Yes, because Source flows both with information and energy to help any suffering person. Reiki healing and intuitive counseling are activated in the presence of need. My anthropology professor said that it is possible for men to nurse an infant. We were amazed by this comment: how could this be so? He said that if there is a situation where there is a crying baby, the mother has died, and no one else is available to feed it, a man's glands can give milk to keep the child from starving. It may take a few days, but it can happen.

Think of yourself as the father who needs to feed the baby. Your compassion will open the milk glands to feed the hungry child. Reiki and intuition flow just like milk, when the need is present, if you are a caring person. It's really quite simple.

LIFELONG INTUITIVE AND
PROFESSIONAL READER: LINDA URIE

Linda Urie is a professional intuitive reader and Reiki Master who makes her home outside Doylestown, the county seat of Bucks County, Pennsylvania. All her adult life she has made a living by giving intuitive readings, although she has never advertised. Her reputation for accuracy, insight, and good humor has spread by word of mouth and kept her busy with a dynamic and varied clientele, many of whom also practice Reiki.

Q: What led you to Reiki? Did intuition and synchronicity play any part?

A: What led me to Reiki was definitely a result of synchronicity, as most of my life is. I received Reiki originally from a client, which made me aware that there was actually a system for intuiting physical energy blocks in the body, something I had done all my life by scanning someone's energy through my palm chakras. I took the Reiki classes as a result of curiosity and out of a regard for a repeatable system for recognizing energy blocks and healing them.

Q: Can you recall an early experience with intuition, your own or someone else's?

A: I am a working psychic medium, so intuitions are very big energy for me. I guess my intuitive awareness goes back to maybe five or six years old. I always felt comfortable with this ability.

Q: Did the adults around you support or discourage this ability?

A: Actually, I never spoke about it that I recall. I just assumed that it would be no big deal. I guess I was probably eight or nine years old when I realized that not everyone connected to what was happening in another's energy. In my late teens I discovered that my mother was also an intuitive, although she never discussed it.

It never occurred to me to do anything but utilize my intuitive abilities, although in the course of a lifetime I don't know that I was always able to do that because of my own personal disruptions. I have, however, done intuitive work on a regular basis for some twenty years now.

Q: When you were attuned to Reiki, did you notice an immediate increase in intuitive abilities or was this a skill that developed with practice?

A: What I noticed was a clearer sense of what was going on not only in another's physical body but also in the emotional body, and an easier pathway to that. I saw Reiki as a positive adjunct to things that I already did. My communications about intuitive impressions have always been very open and very blessed.

Q: Did your Reiki Master provide you with any instruction in how to work with intuition when impressions came up while you did Reiki?

A: Yes, she did. I recall her saying just to sit with an impression until I was clear about what it was, and then I would know intuitively whether to pass this information on or not. I'm sure she gave more detailed instructions, although I don't recall them. Again, I came to her classes with a clearly developed intuitive sense.

Q: Has your intuition become stronger and more helpful since you learned Reiki?

A: I'm not sure if it has become stronger, but during Reiki sessions it is much more focused and specific on the Reiki process.

Q: What was your Reiki Master training like?

A: My Master attunement was in 1997. I spent that year, 1996 to 1997, studying how to use the Usui Reiki system. My Reiki Master was thorough in her teaching.

Q: Have you taught Reiki?

A: I am not active in teaching yet, although it is a definite possibility for the future. And certainly when I do teach I will speak at length to my students about intuition, the intuitive side of self, and how it enhances not only Reiki but everything in life.

Q: How does intuition support you when you offer a Reiki client treatment?

A: I think you can be very clear about whether or not this person is in a space to hear the spoken words, or whether it is better to just quietly support some things that need to be cleared. Not every recipient of Reiki is in an emotional or spiritual space to hear whatever impressions you get, but I think intuition is pretty clear about those to whom you can speak and not.

Q: Can you give an example of how receiving an intuitive impression as you treated yourself with Reiki has helped you?

A: I think that specific parts of the body can speak to specific life issues. I am often drawn to quiet the self through Reiki for sleep disturbances and joint-pain issues. It seems pretty clear why these things occur where they do for me, and Reiki certainly is the preferred delivery system for clearance.

Q: Do you have any specific comments or suggestions for those Reiki practitioners who would like to become more intuitively guided in their practices?

A: I think Reiki is a blessing in its simplicity. I think it is a gift. I am gratified to see how quickly it is growing and how much it has become a part of not only the spiritual community and energetic community, but the medical community as well. It tells me that humanity in general is ready to be more balanced. Reiki practice has added a spectrum to the work that I do that is a blessing, not only to others but to me. In my experience as a lifetime empath and medium, Reiki has brought a sense of process to healing energy, something that I focus much more on since my attunements. Along with awareness and information comes that delivery system, if you will, for healing and for helping people realize that there is another level of existence here—an energetic level.

Be quiet enough and still enough inside to trust what you get. Be in a space where you can sit with it quietly until you are sure of what you are hearing, whether it is spoken or not. Be an observer in what unfolds for the person that you are working on.

SUGGESTIONS FOR PRACTITIONERS

Talk to fellow practitioners and teachers to discover the fascinating and intimately close relationship between intuition and Reiki. While some will believe that they have come to Reiki through conventional means, others will have interesting stories to tell that acknowledge the importance of inner guidance and "external" signs—synchronicities. In addition, by opening up a dialogue with others, you create an opportunity for yourself and others in your Reiki community to continue learning about intuitive Reiki on an ongoing basis.

NOW YOU

If you feel guided to do so, create a safe learning space for you and other practitioners to gather on a weekly, biweekly, or monthly basis to support one another in exploring the nature of intuition, its value in spiritual development, and its use in Reiki practice. Encourage everyone to share their early memories of experiences with intuition and to describe their own responses and the reactions of family members and friends. Help one another discover that the reward for such honest expression of feeling is emotional and mental healing and release from self-doubt.

Follow discussion time with practice time at the table, so that you can experiment with others in your community using the traditional Western and Japanese intuitive Reiki techniques described in this book. When you have developed a sense of competence with these techniques, discuss how to integrate them into your professional Reiki practice.

Finally, experiment with using not only your Reiki hands to listen, but your whole Reiki-charged being, using the techniques for intuitive reading described in chapter 14, "At a Reiki and Intuition Workshop." Enjoy the opportunity to practice using Reiki in "new" ways—by reading a photograph or an inanimate object or drawing someone's aura.

Remember always that Reiki is given to us for the purpose of bringing healing, enlightenment, and empowerment. Be grateful. Be patient and devoted to service. Be glad to practice Reiki and share its many blessings of healing with others. Offer intuitive guidance only on those occasions when it arises on the flow of Reiki energy and you are guided by Spirit to do so. Enjoy the light of Reiki shining within you, the peace of Reiki quieting your mind, and the love of Reiki calling forth and deepening the love within your heart.

APPENDIX 1:
REIKI ORGANIZATIONS

Many traditional Usui method Reiki practitioners and teachers are not affiliated with any formal organization, yet the Usui Reiki Ryoho Gakkai, the Reiki learning society in Japan, has supported generations of practitioners in their spiritual growth and development. Those who are intent on following their own guidance may not feel the need for such support, but for those who wish to explore the benefits of joining an organization, consider the following:

The Reiki Alliance
204 N. Chestnut Street
Kellogg, ID 83837
(208) 783-3535
www.reikialliance.org / info@reikialliance.com

Focus: Spiritual leadership; fellowship; preservation of original Usui Reiki methods of healing and instruction as taught by Hawayo Takata

The Radiance Technique International Association, Inc.
P.O. Box 40570
St. Petersburg, FL 33743-0570
(727) 347-2106
www.trtia.org / trtia@aol.com

Focus: Teaching of The Radiance Technique; peace projects

The International Center for Reiki Training
21421 Hilltop Street, Unit #28
Southfield, MI 48034
(800) 332-8112; local: (248) 948-8112
www.reiki.org / center@reiki.org

Focus: Community education; teaching of non-traditional Usui Reiki, Usui-Tibetan Reiki, and Karuna Reiki

Reiki Outreach International
Ann Thevenin, Director
P.O. Box 191156
San Diego, CA 92119-1156
www.annieo.com/reikioutreach/index.htm / ann@annieo.com

Focus: Humanitarian service; world healing

International Association of Reiki
14823 Mills Park Lane
Cypress, Texas 77429
(281) 373-3675
www.wisechoices.com/reiki.asp

Focus: Teaching Usui Reiki; developing uniform teaching standards

International Association of Reiki Professionals
P.O. Box 6182
Nashua, New Hampshire 03063-6182
(603) 881-8838
www.iarp.org / info@iarp.org

Focus: Supporting practitioners and teachers worldwide; partnering with medical community; promoting spiritual growth and development

The UK Reiki Federation
PO Box 1785
Andover, SP11 OWB
0870 850 2209
www.reikifed.co.uk / enquiry@reikifed.co.uk

Focus: Distance healing; networking; community events

APPENDIX 2:
INTUITION DEVELOPMENT
WORKSHOP PROVIDERS

Reiki practitioners and teachers who wish to hone their intuitive skills to bring to the client treatment table or to use for personal guidance may enjoy taking advantage of opportunities for further training offered by the following organizations and individuals:

Association for Research and Enlightenment (A.R.E.)
215 67th Street
Virginia Beach, VA 23451-2061
(800) 333-4499
www.edgarcayce.org

The Edgar Cayce Institute for Intuitive Studies
215 67th Street
Virginia Beach, VA 23451-2061
(800) 333-4499
www.edgarcayce-intuitionschool.com / intuition@edgarcayce.org

Hay House, Inc.
P.O. Box 5100
Carlsbad, CA 92018-5100
(800) 654-5126
www.hayhouse.com

Intuitive Advantage, Inc.
P. O. Box 4727
Frisco, CO 80443
(970) 668-8300; voice mail: (800) 375-9425
www.intuitiveadvantage.com / info@intuitiveadvantage.com

Linda Schiller-Hanna
7148 Chatham Road
Medina, OH 44256
(330) 725-0597
www.lightworker22.com / linda@lightworker22.com

The Reiki and Intuition Workshop
P.O. Box 1061
Quakertown, PA 18951
www.traditionalreiki.com / amy@traditionalreiki.com

SUGGESTED READING

BOOKS ON REIKI

Barnett, Libby, and Maggie Chambers, with Susan Davidson. *Reiki Energy Medicine: Bringing Healing Touch into Home, Hospital, and Hospice.* Rochester: Healing Arts Press, 1996.

Brown, Fran. *Living Reiki: Takata's Teachings.* Mendocino: LifeRhythm, 1992.

Doi, Hiroshi. *Iyashino Gendai Reiki-ho: Modern Reiki Method for Healing.* Edited by Rick Rivard and Miyuki Iwasaki. Translated by Akiko Kawarai et al. Coquitlam, B.C., Canada: Fraser, 2000.

Haberly, Helen. *Reiki: Hawayo Takata's Story.* Olney: Archedigm, 1990.

Hall, Mari. *Practical Reiki.* London: Thorsens, 2001.

———. *Reiki for the Soul: Ten Doorways to Inner Peace.* London: Thorsens, 2002.

———. *Reiki for the Soul: The Eleventh Doorway.* London: Thorsens, 2006.

———. *Reiki for Common Ailments: A Practical Guide to Healing.* London: Piatkus, 1999.

———. *Reiki: Using Healing Energy for Peace, Joy, Vitality.* New York: Harper Collins, 2002.

Honervogt, Tanmaya. *Inner Reiki: A Practical Guide for Healing and Meditation.* London: Gaia, 2001.

———. *The Power of Reiki: An Ancient Hands-on Healing Technique.* London: Gaia, 1998.

Lubeck, Walter, Frank Arjava Petter, and William Lee Rand. *The Spirit of Reiki: The Complete Handbook of the Reiki System.* Twin Lakes: Lotus Press, 2001.

Narrin, janeAnne. *One Degree Beyond—A Reiki Journey into Energy Medicine: Your 21-Day*

Step-by-Step Guide to Relax, Open and Celebrate. Seattle: Little White Buffalo, 1998.

Petter, Frank Arjava, Tadao Yamaguchi, and Chujiro Hayashi. *Hayashi Reiki Manual: Traditional Japanese Healing Techniques.* Twin Lakes: Lotus Press, 2003.

———— and Dr. Mikao Usui. *The Original Handbook of Dr. Mikao Usui.* Translated by Christine M. Grimm. Twin Lakes: Lotus Press, 1999.

————. *Reiki Fire: New Information about the Origins of the Reiki Power—A Complete Manual.* Twin Lakes: Lotus Light, 1997.

————. *Reiki: The Legacy of Dr. Usui.* Translated by Christine M. Grimm. Twin Lakes: Lotus Light, 1998.

Rand, William. *Reiki, The Healing Touch: First and Second Degree Manual.* Southfield: Vision Publications, 1991.

————. *Reiki for a New Millennium.* New Delhi: Health Harmony, 2001.

————, Frank Arjava Petter, and Walter Lubeck. *The Spirit of Reiki.* Twin Lakes: Lotus press, 2001.

Rivard, Rick R., and Tom Rigler. *Usui Reiki Ryoho: Shoden, Okuden and Shinpiden Japanese Reiki Workshop Manual.* Toronto and Baltimore: Reiki-ho Resources, universal copyright 1999, 2000.

Rowland, Amy Z. *Traditional Reiki for Our Times: Practical Methods for Personal and Planetary Healing.* Rochester: Healing Arts Press, 1998.

Shanti-Gaia, Laurelle. *The Book on Karuna Reiki: Advanced Healing Energy for Our Evolving World.* Sedona: Infinite Light, 2001.

BOOKS ON CREATIVITY

Bryan, Mark, Julia Cameron, and Catherine Allen. *The Artist's Way at Work: Riding the Dragon.* New York: William Morrow, 1998.

Cameron, Julia, and Mark Bryan. *The Artist's Way: A Spiritual Path to Higher Creativity.* New York: Putnam, 1992.

————. *The Vein of Gold: The Journey to Your Creative Heart.* New York: Tarcher/Putnam, 1996.

————. *Walking in This World: The Practical Art of Creativity.* New York: Tarcher/Putnam, 2002.

Maisel, Eric, Ph.D. *Fearless Creating: A Step-by-Step Guide to Starting and Completing Your Work of Art.* New York: Tarcher/Putnam, 1995.

BOOKS ON DREAMWORK

Garfield, Patricia, Ph.D. *Creative Dreaming: Plan and Control Your Dreams to Develop Creativity, Overcome Fears, Solve Problems.* New York: Fireside, 1974, 1995.

LaBerge, Stephen. *Lucid Dreaming: A Concise Guide to Awakening in Your Dreams and in Your Life.* Boulder: Sounds True, 2004.

Moss, Robert. *Conscious Dreaming: A Spiritual Path for Everyday Life.* New York: Three Rivers, 1996.

BOOKS ON JOURNALING

Baldwin, Christina. *Life's Companion: Journal Writing as a Spiritual Quest.* New York: Bantam, 1990.

Breathnach, Sarah Ban. *Simple Abundance: A Daybook of Comfort and Joy.* New York: Time Warner, 1995.

————. *Something More: Excavating Your Authentic Self.* New York: Time Warner, 1998.

DeSalvo, Louise. *Writing as a Way of Healing: How Telling Our Stories Transforms Our Lives.* Boston: Beacon, 1999.

Goldberg, Natalie. *Writing Down the Bones: Freeing the Writer Within.* Boston: Shambala, 1986.

McClanahan, Rebecca. *Write Your Heart Out: Exploring and Expressing What Matters to You.* Cincinnati: Walking Stick, 2001.

Progoff, Ira. *At a Journal Workshop: The Basic Text and Guide for Using the Intensive Journal Process.* New York: Dialogue House, 1975.

BOOKS ON INTUITION AND GUIDANCE

Anderson, George, and Andrew Barone. *Lessons from the Light: Extraordinary Messages of Comfort and Hope from the Other Side.* New York: Berkley, 1999.

Bodine, Echo. *The Gift: Understand and Develop Your Psychic Abilities.* Novato: New World, 2003.

————. *A Still, Small Voice: A Psychic's Guide to Awakening Intuition.* Novato: New World, 2001.

Browne, Sylvia. *Past Lives, Future Healing: A Psychic Reveals the Secrets to Good Health and Great Relationships.* New York: New American Library, 2001.

Choquette, Sonia, Ph.D. *The Psychic Pathway: A Workbook for Reawakening the Voice of Your Soul.* New York: Three Rivers, 1994, 1995.

———. *Your Heart's Desire: Instructions for Creating the Life Your Really Want.* New York: Three Rivers, 1997.

Edward, John. *One Last Time: A Psychic Medium Speaks to Those We Have Loved and Lost.* New York: Berkley, 1998, 1999.

Mark, Barbara, and Trudy Griswold. *Angelspeake: How to Talk with Your Angels.* New York: Simon & Schuster, 1995.

———. *The Angelspeake Book of Prayer and Healing: How to Work with Your Angels.* New York: Simon & Schuster, 1997.

Martin, Angela. *Practical Intuition: Practical Tools for Harnessing the Power of Your Instinct.* New York: Barnes & Noble, 2002.

Myss, Caroline. *Intuitive Power: Your Natural Resources.* CD-ROM. Carlsbad: Hay House, 2004.

Northrup, Christiane, M.D., and Mona Lisa Schulz, M.D., Ph.D. *Igniting Intuition.* CD-ROM. Carlsbad: Hay House, 2005.

Robinson, Lynn A., M.Ed. *Divine Intuition: Your Guide to Creating a Life You Love.* New York: Dorling Kindersley, 2001.

Roads, Michael J. *Talking with Nature: Sharing the Energies and Spirit of Trees, Plants, Birds, and Earth.* Novato: New World, 1985, 1987.

Roman, Sonaya. *Opening to Channel: How to Connect with Your Guide.* Tiburon: Kramer, 1987.

Schulz, Mona Lisa, M.D., Ph.D. *Awakening Intuition: Using Your Mind-Body Network for Insight and Healing.* New York: Harmony, 1998.

Van Praagh, James. *Heaven and Earth: Making the Psychic Connection.* New York: Pocket, 2001.

———. *Talking to Heaven: A Medium's Message of Life After Death.* New York: Dutton, 1997.

Virtue, Doreen, Ph.D. *Divine Guidance: How to Have a Dialogue with God and Your Guardian Angels.* New York: St. Martins, 1998.

———. *Divine Prescriptions: Using Your Sixth Sense—Spiritual Solutions for You and Your Loved Ones.* Los Angeles: Renaissance, 2000.

BOOKS ON THE MIND-BODY CONNECTION

Borysenko, Joan, Ph.D. *Minding the Body, Mending the Mind.* CD-ROM. Carlsbad: Hay House, 2005.

———. *The Power of the Mind to Heal.* Carlsbad: Hay House, 1995.

Capacchione, Lucia, Ph.D. *Living with Feeling: The Art of Emotional Expression.* New York: Tarcher/Putnam, 2001.

Frankl, Victor E. *Man's Search for Meaning.* Boston: Beacon, 1959, 1984.

Hay, Louise. *Heal Your Body: The Mental Causes for Physical Illness and the Metaphysical Way to Overcome Them.* Carlsbad: Hay House, 1982.

———. *You Can Heal Your Life.* Carlsbad: Hay House, 1984.

Pert, Candace, Ph.D. *Molecules of Emotion: Why You Feel the Way You Feel.* New York: Scribner, 1997.

Steadman, Alice. *Who's the Matter with Me?* Marina del Rey: DeVorss, 1966, 1967, 1968.

BOOKS ON PRAYER AND MEDITATION

Braybrooke, Marcus, ed. *The Bridge of Stars: 365 Prayers, Blessings, and Meditations from Around the World.* London: Thorsons, 2001.

Dossey, Larry, M.D. *Healing Words: The Power of Prayer and the Practice of Medicine.* San Francisco: Harper, 1993.

Radha, Swami Sivananda. *The Divine Light Invocation: A Healing Meditation.* Spokane: Timeless, 2001.

Walsch, Neale Donald. *Conversations with God: An Uncommon Dialogue (Book 1).* New York: Putnam, 1995.

———. *Conversations with God: An Uncommon Dialogue (Book 2).* Charlottesville: Hampton Roads, 1997.

———. *Conversations with God: An Uncommon Dialogue (Book 3).* Charlottesville: Hampton Roads, 1998.